OXFORD HANDBOOKS IN EMERGENCY MEDICINE
Series Editors   R. N. Illingworth, C. E. Robertson, and A. D. Redmond

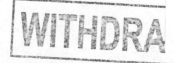

OXFORD HANDBOOKS IN EMERGENCY MEDICINE

This series will cover topics of interest to all Accident and Emergency staff. The books are aimed at junior doctors and casualty nurses. Each book starts with an introduction to the topic, including epidemiology where appropriate. The clinical presentation and the immediate practical management of common conditions is described in detail, so that the casualty officer or nurse is able to deal with the problem on the spot. A specific course of action is recommended for each situation, and alternatives discussed.

Accidents and Emergencies in Children

Rosemary J. Morton FRCP, FRCS, FFAEM
Consultant in Accident and Emergency Medicine,
Manchester Royal Infirmary, Manchester

and

Barbara M. Phillips FRCP, FFAEM
Consultant Paediatrician in Accident and Emergency,
Booth Hall Children's Hospital, Manchester

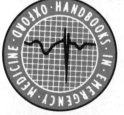

Oxford • New York • Tokyo
OXFORD UNIVERSITY PRESS

Oxford   New York
Athens   Auckland   Bangkok   Bombay
Calcutta   Cape Town   Dar es Salaam   Delhi
Florence   Hong Kong   Istanbul   Karachi
Kuala Lumpur   Madras   Madrid   Melbourne
Mexico City   Nairobi   Paris   Singapore
Taipei   Tokyo   Toronto
and associated companies in
Berlin   Ibadan

Oxford is a trade mark of Oxford University Press

Published in the United States
by Oxford University Press Inc., New York

First edition published 1992
Second edition published 1996
© Rosemary J. Morton and Barbara M. Phillips, 1992, 1996

A catalogue record for this book is available from the British Library

Library of Congress Cataloging in Publication Data
ISBN 0 19 262720 1 (Hbk)
ISBN 0 19 262719 8 (Pbk)

Typeset by Footnote Graphics, Warminster, Wilts
Printed in Great Britain by
Biddles Ltd, Guildford and King's Lynn

For Bryony and Robert
and
for Ruth and Rachel

Preface to the first edition

We have written this book to help Accident and Emergency senior house officers, who may have no postgraduate paediatric experience, to manage the wide variety of paediatric patients who attend their departments.

Emphasis has been placed on the emergency management of serious illness and injury, and on the management of common problems.

Indications for referral to paediatric and other specialists are clearly made. However, in many instances further management is also described both for readers studying for the Accident and Emergency Fellowship examination and in case paediatric help is otherwise occupied!

Although efforts have been made to ensure the accuracy of drug dosage, readers should consult the *British National Formulary* before prescribing.

Our thanks go to our teachers over years of medical practice and to our many colleagues, patients, and families from whom we have learnt how to care for children. Particular thanks are offered to our paediatric colleagues who have contributed helpful criticisms from their own specialist expertise—Tim David, Jon Couriel (also permission to use Table 16.1), David Evans, Mike Clarke, John Keen, Raine Roberts, Frank Bamford, Victor Miller, Peter Davenport, and Sheila Stainthorpe (permission to modify Table 2.2).

The guidance of Robin Illingworth, the series editor, and the support of Oxford University Press were invaluable.

Finally, we thank John Coffey for the drawings, Jennifer Loxley for her patience with countless manuscript revisions, and our families for tolerating the time spent away from them.

1991   R.J.M.
Manchester   B.M.P.

Contents

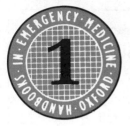

CHAPTER 1

Children in the Accident and Emergency department

Facilities for children and their families

Between 20 and 30 per cent of attenders at District General Hospital Accident and Emergency (A & E) departments are children under 16 years old. In England and Wales there are more than two million child attenders at A & E departments annually. There is a disproportionately high number of attenders under five years of age.

It is sometimes considered that because children are small they require a smaller provision of space in hospital buildings than do adults. In fact the opposite is true. Children attending A & E departments are usually accompanied by at least one adult, and often siblings, prams, or pushchairs.

The requirements in Box 1.1 are supported by the joint statement on children's A & E attendances produced in 1988 by the British Paediatric Association, the British Association of Paediatric Surgeons, and the Casualty Surgeons Association (now the British Association for Accident and Emergency Medicine).

A separate resuscitation area for children is not appropriate for most A & E departments, but equipment and drugs for children should be easily identifiable and available.

Box 1.1 Minimum requirements for children in A & E

- Separate triage and waiting area with play facilities.
- Separate treatment area suitably decorated and equipped.
- Private room for distressed parents.
- At least one RSCN trained nurse on the staff.
- A consultant paediatrician to have responsibility for liaison with the consultant in A & E medicine concerning general arrangements for children.
- A liaison health visitor to facilitate communication between the department and the community.

Categories of paediatric problems in A & E

- **Trauma   Medical   Surgical   Behavioural/psychiatric problems**

Trauma

Injured children account for the majority of attendances (60–70 per cent). Most will have relatively minor injuries, but a few will have suffered major blunt or, more rarely, penetrating injury, or severe burns or scalds, or will have been seriously poisoned.

Accidents are the most common cause of death in children over one year old in the United Kingdom. Each year, about 700 children die as a result of accidents, and about 10 000 become permanently disabled. About 20 per cent of children's admissions to hospital are the result of accidents.

Medical

Fifteen to twenty per cent of attenders have medical problems. These will range from the seriously ill child with convulsions, collapse, or respiratory difficulty, to patients who have conditions usually treated by their general practitioner (GP). In this latter group are children who have been treated by their GP but whose parents want a 'second opinion', children whose illness is not improving as quickly as their parents expect, and children whose parents fear that they are seriously ill. Children under five years old, and especially children under two, predominate in the medical attenders.

Surgical

A smaller percentage of patient's have non-traumatic surgical problems, such as irritable hip. Perthes' disease, appendicitis, hernia, etc.

Behavioural/psychiatric problems

A small number of children, usually adolescents, attend with symptoms related to drug, alcohol, or solvent abuse, or following self-poisoning attempts.

The problem of **child abuse** may be found throughout the whoel spectrum of A & E attenders.

The child in the A & E department

• **Triage   The importance of play   The approach to the child and parents   Treatment and procedures   Information   Liaison with other departments**

Triage

Patients are assessed on arrival by an experienced nurse who decides if they require urgent treatment or can safely wait. Children are usually given a high priority. It is important to remember that seriously ill babies can be presented in their parents' arms as apparently 'walking wounded.'

The importance of play

A & E attendance when acutely injured or ill is a frightening introduction to hospital for a child. Play reduces anxiety in an unfamiliar situation, as it is through play that children learn and express themselves. Children's cooperation can be more easily secured if, while waiting, they are distracted by playing and, when examined or undergoing procedures, the element of play is introduced.

The approach to the child and parents

When first meeting a family, introduce yourself, know the child's name, and ascertain if the accompanying adults are the child's parents. Talk to the child even if he is not old enough to understand—even babies love being talked to. Praise encourages cooperation during the examination: for example, 'How good you are being'.

The examination of children, especially young ones, often does not proceed in an ordered fashion and one must be opportunistic while examining. Leave unpleasant procedures, such as throat or rectal examination, until last.

Treatment and procedures

To minimize anxiety both for the child and the parent it is most important that the parent accompanies the child through all treatments and procedures. In some cases this may even include treatment in the resuscitation room. A parent who has not accompanied the child to the resuscitation room must be brought back to be with the child again as soon as the emergency situation is under control. Children should be given a clear explanation appropriate to their age before the start of any procedure.

Information

Leaflets detailing instructions for parents, problems to look out for, and information on who to contact in the event of concern are very useful for parents of children who are discharged from the department. Appropriate translations should be available for non-English-speaking families.

Liaison with other departments

Close liaison is needed between the A & E department and the paediatric, anaesthetic, orthopaedic, and surgical departments in particular. This liaison will be facilitated if there is feedback from other departments on the progress of children who have been admitted to hospital and if joint audit meetings can be held.

GPs should receive information on all of their patients who

have attended the local A & E department. Health visitors are informed after each child's attendance.

Recognition of children with potentially serious illness

It is often difficult in the early stages of illness to differentiate the child with serious illness from one with a mild self-limiting disease. Two small groups of children need to be differentiated from the larger group with benign self-limiting disease.

(1) the child with a severe form of a common, often benign disease, for example gastroenteritis or pneumonia;

(2) the child with early serious disease always requiring hospital treatment, for example meningitis or pyloric stenosis.

In addition to history and examination, the clinical assessment of children includes observation to assess whether they look 'ill' or not. There are four steps in the initial assessment of the unwell child:

- history
- observation
- examination
- investigation.

1. History—In addition to disease-specific symptoms, such as cough, breathing difficulties, vomiting, diarrhoea, convulsions, cyanosis, etc., the history of an infant's alertness, interaction with his environment, and overall activity is important when assessing the presence of serious illness. Other useful non-specific symptoms are taking less than half the ususal amount of fluid and passing less urine than usual in the previous 24 hours. These general symptoms are often not mentioned by the parent who will usually concentrate on the more graphic symptoms, such as cough, vomiting, or diarrhoea. Careful questioning of the parent is necessary to elicit this aspect of the history.

2. Observation—Before a systematic examination of the patient there should be a period of observation (often while taking the history) for evidence as to whether the child looks 'ill' or not. The child should be on the patient's lap, or wherever he seems happy, and observation should be made of the following.

- Alertness—a well child will look around at his environment but an ill child will be uninterested or irritable.
- Interaction with parents—does he respond to his parents, playing if happy, or is he easily distracted when crying? A child who is ill will be less easily interested or distracted than one who is well.
- Interaction with the doctor—a baby will respond to eye contact, smile if he is old enough, or reach out for a proffered toy, but the unwell baby will show a lack of interest.
- State of wakefulness—the well baby will wake up quickly when stimulated if asleep, and if awake will stay alert. The unwell baby takes some time to wake up and becomes drowsy easily.

3. Examination—specific physical signs of disease are referred to in the relevant chapters.

4. Investigations—recommended investigations can be found in the relevant chapters.

A score called 'Baby Check' has been devised and tested for use in babies under six months old. It has been designed to help parents to differentiate between the non-specific symptoms of mild disease and early serious disease by means of 19 scored symptoms and signs (see reference 5).

The febrile child

The infant child with a fever is often presented for medical attention early in the disease when specific clinical diagnosis is difficult.

First, assess the child's overall condition. *Seek urgent paediatric help with the febrile child who is drowsy, unresponsive, or pale*, or who has a purpuric rash. He may have septicaemia (p. 34, 35), meningitis (p. 216/220), pyelonephritis or a severe episode of a more common infection such as gastroenteritis (p. 188).

The history may be helpful in suggesting a focus for the illness; for example, there may have been diarrhoea, a cough, a painful throat, or earache.

Thorough examination will reveal the infectious focus in some children. Common causes of fever are

- colds (p. 168)
- tonsillitis (p. 170)
- pharyngitis (p. 170)
- otitis media (p. 169)
- the exanthems, e.g. measles (p. 233)

The following causes are less common but should be considered in a child with unexplained fever:

- meningtis (p. 216, 220)
- septicaemia (p. 34)
- urinary tract infection (p. 202)
- pneumonia (p. 176)
- peritonitis (p. 194)
- osteomyelitis/septic arthritis (p. 119)

The white cell count is generally unhelpful in the assessment of the febrile child, although occasionally it may point to a specific diagnosis, for example atypical mononuclear cells in glandular fever.

Infectious diseases not endemic in the UK should be considered in febrile recent travellers.

Children for whom no cause for fever can be found and those who are unwell should be referred to the paediatric team.

Further reading

1. British Paediatric Association, British Association of Paediatric Surgeons, Casualty Surgeons Association (1988). *Joint statement on children's attendances at Accident & Emergency departments.* British Paediatric Association, London.
2. Royal College of Nursing (1989). *Nursing children in Accident & Emergency Departments: guidelines for children and the family.* Royal College of Nursing, London.
3. National Association for the Welfare of Children in Hospital (1990). *NAWCH quality review: setting standards for children in health care.* National Association for the Welfare of Children in Hospital, London (now Action for Sick Children).
4. Child Accident Prevention Trust (1989). *Basic principles of child*

accident prevention: a guide to action. Child Accident Prevention Trust, London.

5. Morley, C.J., Thornton, A.J., Cole, T.J., and Hewson, P.H. (1991). Interpreting the symptoms and signs of illness in infants. In *Recent advances in paediatrics*, No. 4 (ed. T.J. David), pp. 137–55. Churchill Livingstone, Edinburgh (description of 'Baby Check' score).

CHAPTER 2

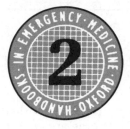

Cardiopulmonary resuscitation and the seriously ill child

Key points in cardiopulmonary resuscitation

1 Respiratory and/or circulatory failure are the usual causes of cardiac arrest in children.

2 Airway control and ventilation with 100 per cent oxygen are of prime importance.

3 Venous or intraosseous access must be gained as soon as possible for circulatory support and administration of drugs.

4 Earlier recognition and treatment of imminent respiratory and circulatory failure will improve outcome.

5 Overwhelming infection is a frequent precursor of collapse, especially in infancy. After initial resuscitation early consideration should be given to the use of intravenous broad-spectrum antibiotics.

Introduction

- **Aetiology of cardiac arrests   Outcome   Summoning help**

Aetiology of cardiac arrests

Cardiac arrests in children are rarely due to primary cardiac problems. Most are the result of hypoxia and some are caused by circulatory failure (Fig. 2.1). The mode of death in sudden infant death syndrome (p. 259) is unknown.

Outcome

The outcome of respiratory arrest alone should initially be good, and long-term survival depends on the underlying

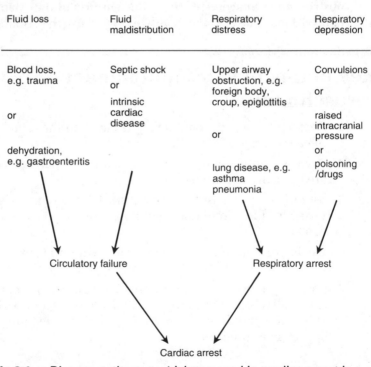

Fluid loss	Fluid maldistribution	Respiratory distress	Respiratory depression
Blood loss, e.g. trauma

or

dehydration, e.g. gastroenteritis | Septic shock

or

intrinsic cardiac disease | Upper airway obstruction, e.g. foreign body, croup, epiglottitis

or

lung disease, e.g. asthma pneumonia | Convulsions

or

raised intracranial pressure

or

poisoning /drugs |

Circulatory failure   Respiratory arrest

Cardiac arrest

Fig 2.1 • Disease pathways which may end in cardiac arrest in childhood.

pathology. However, the outcome of cardiac arrest in children is less good than that in adults. Many cardiac arrests in adults result from ventricular fibrillation; the heart rhythm and output can often be restored by prompt defibrillation. However, in children most cardiac arrests are caused by hypoxia or shock and the cardiac rhythm is usually asystole. In children, the heart is usually healthy and withstands hypoxia and acidosis for longer than the brain. By the time cardiac arrest has occurred, the injury to the brain and other organs may be too severe to permit recovery even if the heart is restarted.

The worst outcome is in children who arrive apnoeic and pulseless at an A & E department. These children have a poor chance of intact neurological survival. There has often been a prolonged period of hypoxia and ischaemia before the start of adequate cardiopulmonary resuscitation. Earlier recognition of seriously ill children and paediatric cardiopulmonary resuscitation (CPR) training for ambulance personnel and the public could improve the outcome for these children.

Summoning help

When a child with a suspected respiratory or cardiac arrest is brought into the A & E department, an immediate emergency call should be made for the paediatrician and the anaesthetist. The A & E staff must start resuscitation. Table 2.1 gives a list of suggested personnel and their initial tasks. One member of the team must assume leadership. A rapid history should be obtained from parents or ambulance personnel and relayed to the resuscitation team. Such information is vital to

Table 2.1 • Arrest team personnel

Personnel	Suggested initial task
Anaesthetist	Airway and breathing management
A & E SHO	Cardiac compression
Paediatric SHO and/or Registrar	IV access and drugs
Nurse 1	Assist anaesthetist with airway and breathing
Nurse 2	Drug and IV fluid preparation
Nurse 3	Monitors and charts
Nurse 4	Liaison with parents

Table 2.2 •

				Prem.	Newborn
		Age			
		Average weight		2 kg	3 kg
				4.5 lb	7 lb
		ETT diameter		2.5–3 mm	3 mm
		Oral ETT length		8.5 cm	9.5 cm
		Nasal ETT length		10 cm	11 cm
		Chest drain F (Ch) gauge		8	8
		Urinary catheter F gauge		3.5	5
		Minimum artificial ventilation rate		40/min	40/min
		Defibrillator charge			
		1st and 2nd—2 J/kg		4 J6 J	
		3rd–4 J/kg		8 J	10 J
Drug	*Dose*	*Concentration*	*Route*		
Atropine	20 µg/kg	600 µg/ml	IV or ETT	0.17 ml	0.17 ml
Adrenaline first dose	10 µg/kg	1:10 000	IV or ETT	0.2 ml	0.3 ml
Adrenaline second dose	100 µg/kg	1:1000	IV	0.2 ml	0.3 ml
Sodium bicarbonate	1 mmol/kg	8.4% (1 mmol/ml)	IV	2 ml	3 ml
Lignocaine	1 mg/kg	1%	IV or ETT	0.2 ml	0.3 ml
Calcium chloride	10 mg/kg	10%	IV	0.2 ml	0.3 ml
Frusemide	1 mg/kg	20 mg/2 ml	IV	0.2 ml	0.3 ml
Mannitol	500 mg/kg	10%	IV	10 ml	15 ml
		20%	IV	5 ml	7.5 ml
Dopamine	5 µg/kg/min	Dissolve 150 mg dopamine in 500 ml dextrose 5%	IV	2 ml/h	3 ml/h
Dobutamine	10 µg/kg/min	Dissolve 300 mg dobutamine in 500 ml dextrose 5%	IV	2 ml/h	3 ml/h
		Age		Prem.	Newborn
		Average weight		2 kg	3 kg

ETT, endotracheal tube. Equipment sizes are only a guide. A size larger or smaller may be required. ETT dose is different (see text). All IV doses may be given 10.

the resuscitation effort; for example, if the child has had pro-fuse diarrhoea, volume replacement is especially important.

Airway and breathing management, cardiac compression, and IV access and drug administration must proceed simultaneously. Patient observations and drugs must be documented.

Table 2.2 shows sizes of equipment needed and doses of drugs to be used in CPR.

1 m	2 m	3 m	6 m	1 yr	2 yr	3 yr	5 yr	7 yr	10 yr	15 yr
4 kg	4.5 kg	5 kg	8 kg	10 kg	13 kg	15 kg	18 kg	23 kg	30 kg	40+ kg
9 lb	10 lb	12 lb	17 lb	22 lb	29 lb	33 lb	40 lb	50 lb	66 lb	88+ lb
3 mm	3 mm	3.5 mm	4 mm	4 mm	4.5 mm	5 mm	5 m	6.5 mm	7.5 mm	7.5 mm
10 cm	10 cm	10.5 cm	11 cm	12 cm	13 cm	13.5 cm	14 cm	16 cm	18.5 cm	19 cm
11.5 cm	11.5 cm	12 cm	12.5 cm	14.5 cm	15 cm	16 cm	16.8 cm	18 cm	19 cm	20 cm
8	8	10	10	10	12	14	16	18	20	24
5	5	8	8	8	10	10	12	12	16	16
40/min	40/min	40/min	30/min	30/min	30/min	30/min	30/min	25/min	25/min	25/min
8 J	9 J	10 J	15 J	20 J	25 J	30 J	40 J	50 J	60 J	100 J
16 J	18 J	20 J	30 J	40 J	50 J	60 J	80 J	100 J	120 J	200 J
0.17 ml	0.17 ml	0.2 ml	0.25 ml	0.35 ml	0.5 ml	0.5 ml	0.6 ml	0.8 ml	1 ml	1 ml
0.4 ml	0.45 ml	0.5 ml	0.8 ml	1 ml	1.3 ml	1.5 ml	1.8 ml	2.5 ml	3 ml	4 ml
0.4 ml	0.45 ml	0.5 ml	0.8 ml	1 ml	1.3 ml	1.5 ml	1.8 ml	2.5 ml	3 ml	4 ml
4 ml	4.5 ml	5 ml	8 ml	10 ml	13 ml	15 ml	18 ml	23 ml	30 ml	40 ml
0.4 ml	0.5 ml	0.5 ml	0.8 ml	1 ml	1.3 ml	1.5 ml	2 ml	2.5 ml	3 ml	4 ml
0.4 ml	0.5 ml	0.5 ml	0.8 ml	1 ml	1.3 ml	1.5 ml	2 ml	2.5 ml	3 ml	4 ml
0.4 ml	0.4 ml	0.5 ml	0.8 ml	1 ml	1.3 ml	1.5 ml	2 ml	2.5 ml	3 ml	4 ml
20 ml	22 ml	25 ml	35 ml	50 ml	65 ml	75 ml	100 ml	125 ml	150 ml	200 ml
10 ml	11 ml	12 ml	17 ml	25 ml	32 ml	37 ml	50 ml	62 ml	75 ml	100 ml
4 ml/h	4.5 ml/h	5 ml/h	8 ml/h	10 ml/h	13 ml/h	15 ml/h	18 ml/h	23 ml/h	30 ml/h	40 ml/h
4 ml/h	4.5 ml/h	5 ml/h	8 ml/h	10 ml/h	13 ml/h	15 ml/h	18 ml/h	23 ml/h	30 ml/h	40 ml/h
1 m	2 m	3 m	6 m	1 yr	2 yr	3 yr	5 yr	7 yr	10 yr	15 yr
4 kg	4.5 kg	5 kg	8 kg	10 kg	13 kg	15 kg	18 kg	23 kg	30 kg	40+ kg

Paediatric resuscitation procedure

**Basic life support   Advanced life support   Circulation
Drugs in CPR and post-resuscitation management
Monitoring in CPR**

Basic life support

Assessment of responsiveness The initial assessment of responsiveness involves asking the child 'Are you alright?'

Table 2.3 • Equipment for the paediatric resuscitation area

1. Airway
   - Oropharyngeal airway sizes 000, 00, 0, 1, 2, 3, 4
   - Endotracheal tubes sizes 2.5, 3.0, 3.5, 4.0, 4.5, 5.0, 5.5, 6.0, 6.5, 7.0, 7.5 uncuffed and 7.5 cuffed
   - Oxygen masks for facial oxygen
   - Laryngoscopes
     Neonatal, e.g. Wisconsin type
     Intermediate, e.g. Robertshaw
     Adult, e.g. Macintosh
   - Inflating bag, e.g. Laerdal, Ambu (with reservoirs)
     240 ml infant size
     500 ml child size
     1600 ml adult size
   - Transparent cuffed masks for inflating bags
     Infant—circular 01, 1, 2
     Child—shaped to nose 2, 3
     Adult—shaped to nose 4, 5
   - Connections, e.g. Portex type
   - Magill forceps
   - Yankauer sucker
   - Tracheal catheters
   - Ayre's T-piece anaesthetic circuit
   - Needle cricothyrotomy set
2. ECG monitor with defibrillator (with paediatric paddles)
3. Automatic blood pressure monitor (with infant and child-sized cuffs)
4. Pulse oximeter (with infant and child-sized probes)
5. Intravenous access requirements, e.g.
   - Jelco   18–24 gauge
   - Venflon   18–24 gauge
   - Medicut   18–24 gauge
   - Butterfly   18–25 gauge
   - Intraosseous infusion needles 16–18 gauge
   - Graduated burette
   - Intravenous giving sets
   - Syringes 1–50 ml sizes
6. Intravenous drip monitoring device, e.g. Imed
7. Cut-down set
8. Dextrostix or BM Stix
9. Chest drain set 8–28 F (Ch) sizes
10. Urinary catheters 8–18 F sizes
11. Seldinger percutaneous cannulation set
12. Nasogastric tubes 3.5–16 F sizes

and gently shaking him or her by one shoulder. Children too young to talk and older children who are frightened are unlikely to reply, but may make some sound or open their eyes to the assessor's voice. In any victim where trauma is a possibility, the neck and spine should be immobilized during the manoeuvre by placing one hand firmly on the forehead and shaking one of the child's arms gently.

Airway In many unconscious children the airway may be obstructed by the tongue falling back and blocking the pharynx. Correction of this obstruction can result in recovery without further intervention. An attempt should be made to open the airway using the head-tilt–chin-lift manoeuvre. The rescuer places a hand on the child's forehead and applies pressure to tilt the head back gently. The degrees of tilt are 'neutral' in the infant and 'sniffing' in the child. The fingers of the other hand are then placed under the chin which is lifted upwards. Care must be taken not to injure the soft tissue by gripping too hard. This movement may close the child's mouth, and therefore it may be necessary to use the thumb of the same hand to part the lips slightly. The airway's patency should then be assessed by **looking** for chest movement, **listening** for breath sounds, and **feeling** for exhaled breath. If this airway-opening manoeuvre has been unsuccessful or is contraindicated because the patient has been a trauma victim (see Chapter 3), then the jaw-thrust manoeuvre can be performed. Two or three fingers are placed under the child's mandible bilaterally and the jaw is lifted forwards. The success or failure of the manoeuvre is then assessed by the same look, listen, and feel technique as just described.

If appropriate, an oropharyngeal airway can be inserted into the mouth, concave side up, and then, when it is over the tongue, turned over to slide into place. This will maintain the open airway by preventing the tongue from pressing back on the posterior pharyngeal wall. In infants the oropharyngeal airway should be inserted convex side up using a tongue depressor to avoid pushing the tongue into the pharynx.

Breathing If the airway-opening techniques described above do not result in the child's starting to breathe, breathing support should be commenced.

Initially, five rescue breaths are given. In hospital these can be given with self-inflating bag and mask using oxygen as the inflating gas. The appropriate sized inflating bag and mask should be used, and it is important to ensure a good airtight seal between the mask and the child's face. An oxygen reservoir is necessary for high oxygen concentration.

If the chest does not rise then the airway is not clear. The usual cause is failure to open the airway by the techniques discussed above. Therefore the first thing to do is to readjust the head-tilt–chin-lift position or the jaw-thrust position and try again. Further failure to effect air entry should give rise to the suspicion that a foreign body may be present (see p. 148, 185).

Adequacy of ventilation should be assessed by looking for chest expansion.

Circulation   Once the initial five rescue breaths have been given the circulation should be assessed.

Cardiac arrest is recognized by the absence of a central pulse for five seconds. In older children the carotid artery in the neck can be palpated. However, in infants the neck is generally short and fat and the carotid artery may be difficult to feel. Therefore the brachial artery in the medical aspect of the antecubital fossa or the femoral artery at the groin should be felt.

If the pulse is absent for five seconds or is inadequate (less than 60 beats/minute in infants), chest compressions are required. If the pulse is present and at an adequate rate but apnoea continues, breathing support must be continued until spontaneous respiration resumes.

For good chest compressions, the child must be placed lying flat on his or her back on a hard surface. The area for compression in infants is found by imagining a line between the nipples and compressing over the sternum one finger breadth below this line. Two fingers should be used to compress the chest to a depth of approximately 1.5–2.5 cm. Alternatively, infant chest compression can be achieved by using the hand-encircling technique. The infant is held with both the rescuer's hands encircling the chest, and the thumbs are placed over the correct part of the sternum to carry out compression.

In small children the area of compression is one finger breadth above the xiphisternum. The heel of one hand is used to compress the sternum to a depth of approximately 2.5–3.5 cm.

In older children the area of compression is two finger breadths above the xiphisternum, and the heels of both hands are used to compress the sternum to a depth of 3–4.5 cm depending on the size of the child.

A ratio of five compressions to one ventilation is maintained, and this cycle should be repeated 20 times per minute whatever the age of the child.

Advanced Life Support

In the pulseless infant or child, once a patent airway with adequate respiration is established in conjunction with effective chest compressions, the arrest rhythm must be diagnosed and appropriate advanced life support undertaken.

Chest electrodes should be attached to the patient and the ECG appearance studied. Check that there are no artefacts, caused by a loose wire or disconnected electrode for example, and if necessary turn up the gain on the ECG monitor.

Airway and breathing Although it is possible to maintain adequate ventilation through the bag–valve–mask system, endotracheal intubation secures the airway, can be a route for drug administration, and is necessary if ventilation is to be prolonged.

Endotracheal intubation technique The manoeuvre should be proceeded by bag-and-mask ventilation with 100 per cent oxygen for at least a minute to pre-oxygenate the patient. In the emergency situation there is no need to cut the endotracheal tube to the recommended length for the child's age. When the laryngoscope is passed, an assistant should stand at the child's right-hand side with a wide-bore suction catheter and prepared endotracheal tube. Upward thyroid cartilage pressure may improve the view of the larynx. The laryngoscope is used to lift the base of the tongue forward to expose and illuminate the epiglottis and vocal cords. The tube is passed between the vocal cords. Intubation attempts should be limited to 30 seconds, and then the child should be reoxygenated by bag and mask before the next attempt. When the endotracheal tube is in place, connect the bag and ventilate. Check the tube's position and adequacy of ventilation by looking for chest movement and by listening for air entry with a stethoscope in both axillae and over the abdomen. If only one lung is inflating, then the tube may be down one of the main bronchi. It should be pulled back a short distance and auscultation should occur again. If there are doubts about the positioning or patency of the endotracheal tube, it should be removed and the patient again oxygenated by bag and mask before a further attempt.

In the absence of a chart showing the appropriate sized tube for different ages (Table 2.2) a useful formula for estimating the size of tube is 'age over 4 plus 4' for children over the age of one year. Neonates usually require a 3–3.5 mm tube, although pre-term infants may need one of a smaller size. Another useful guideline is to use a tube of about the same diameter as the child's little finger or of a size that will just fit into his nostril.

Circulation

Asystole This is the most common arrest rhythm in children. The response of the young heart to prolonged hypoxia or acidosis is progressive bradycardia leading to asystole.

The protocol for drug use in asystole is shown in Fig. 2.2. Before the administration of any drug, the patient must be receiving continuous and effective basic life support, have a patent airway, and be adequately ventilated with high concentration oxygen.

Adrenaline improves coronary and cerebral blood flow during chest compressions by peripheral vasoconstriction. The initial intravenous dose is 10 µg/kg (0.1 ml of 1:10 000 solution). This is given through a central line if one is in place, but in the A & E department this is unlikely to be the case. It may be given through a peripheral line if one can be achieved rapidly. However, speed is vital, and if a peripheral cannula cannot be placed within one minute than an introasseous needle should be inserted (see p. 68) and the adrenaline given by this route. If there is an endoctracheal tube in place, this route can be used. Ten times the intravenous dose (i.e. 100 µg/kg) should be injected quickly down the endotracheal tube via a narrow-bore suction catheter and then flushed in with 1–2 ml of normal saline. Intravenous or intraosseous adrenaline should also be flushed in with 5–10 ml of normal saline.

The routine use of alkalizing agents has not been shown to be of benefit. However, children in asystole are very acidotic,

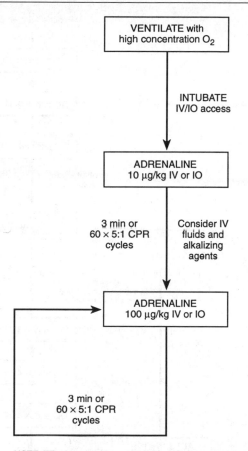

NOTE: ET adrenaline dose × 10 if IV or IO access is not established within 90 seconds.

Fig. 2.2 • Protocol for asystole. Basic life support must be ongoing. ET, endotracheal.

as the cardiac arrest has usually followed a period of respiratory or circulatory collapse. Therefore sodium bicarbonate should be administered in cases where profound acidosis is likely and if the first dose of adrenaline has not produced the return of spontaneous circulation. Similarly, in some cases cardiac arrest may have resulted from circulatory failure, and a 20 ml/kg bolus of fluid (crystalloid or colloid) can be given if there is no response to the initial dose of adrenaline.

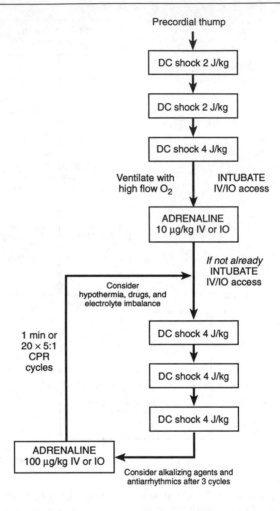

Precordial thump

DC shock 2 J/kg

DC shock 2 J/kg

DC shock 4 J/kg

Ventilate with high flow O$_2$ · INTUBATE IV/IO access

ADRENALINE 10 µg/kg IV or IO

If not already INTUBATE IV/IO access

Consider hypothermia, drugs, and electrolyte imbalance

1 min or 20 × 5:1 CPR cycles

DC shock 4 J/kg

DC shock 4 J/kg

DC shock 4 J/kg

ADRENALINE 100 µg/kg IV or IO

Consider alkalizing agents and antiarrhythmics after 3 cycles

NOTE: ET adrenaline × 10 if IV/IO access is not established within 90 seconds.

Fig 2.3 • Protocol for ventricular fibrillation. Basic life support must be ongoing except when shocks are given.

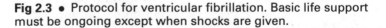

The second bolus of adrenaline is at a dose of ten times that of the first, and if there is still no response to adrenaline with continuing ventilatory support and CPR then further adrenaline is administered every three minutes (60 CPR cycles). The

evidence suggests that the outcome of asystole in children is very poor if there is no response to the second dose of adrenaline.

Ventricular fibrillation   The protocol for ventricular fibrillation management is shown in Fig. 2.3. This arryhthmia is very uncommon in children and is usually precipitated by a recognizable and treatable cause. Without treatment of the underlying cause, the fibrillation may be resistant to conversion.

On identification of fibrillation, electrical defibrillation should be carried out immediately using the dosages in the protocol. Paediatric paddles (4.5 cm) should be used for children under 10 kg. One electrode is placed just below the right clavicle and the other in the left mid-clavicular line at the level of the xiphoid. If paediatric paddles are not available for children of this size, adult paddles may be used, putting one electrode on the front of the chest over the heart and the other on the back of the chest over the heart.

If the first three shocks, given in quick succession, are unsuccessful in converting the rhythm back to normal, the child's coronary and cerebral circulation should be supported as in asystole, with ventilation, chest compressions, and adrenaline. This is followed by a further three shocks while possible causes of the fibrillation are considered and treated. The probable causes are poisoning with drugs such as tricyclic antidepressants, electrolyte imbalance such as hyperkalaemia, and hypothermia. Basic life support should continue at all times apart from when the patient is receiving defibrillation. After every three further DC shocks, an additional dose of adrenaline at the higher level of 100 mcg/kg should be given either intravenously or intraosseously. After three cycles have been unsuccessful, alkalizing agents such as bicarbonate and antiarrhythmics such as lignocaine or bretylium tosylate may be tried. Different paddle positions or another defibrillator could be used if there are doubts about the efficacy of the equipment.

Pulseless electrical activity (electromechanical dissociation)
The protocol for the management of this arrhythmia is shown in Fig. 2.4. Pulseless electrical activity (PEA), also known as electromechanical dissociation, is the absence of a palpable pulse despite the presence of recognizable complexes on the

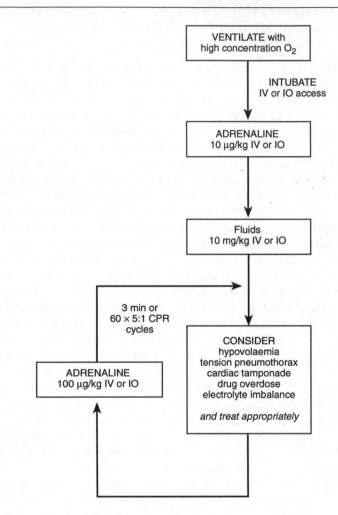

Fig 2.4 • Protocol for electromechanical dissociation.

ECG monitor. Throughout the protocol, the underlying cause should be sought. The most common cause in childhood is severe shock, making the pulse difficult to feel. However, tension pneumothorax and cardiac tamponade should also be considered in the trauma patient. In some patients electrolyte disturbance or the ingestion of a calcium-blocking drug may be a cause, and only in this situation is the use of calcium chloride helpful in cardiac arrest.

Drugs in CPR and post-resuscitation management

Oxygen All patients undergoing CPR initially require 100 per cent oxygen. Potential adverse effects of high oxygen concentration are not a consideration in these circumstances. Bag-and-mask devices give up to 60 per cent delivery with oxygen connected and up to 100 per cent if an oxygen reservoir is added. An Ayre's T-piece bag will deliver 100 per cent oxygen; however, the T-piece circuit is difficult to handle by the inexperienced and is probably best left for the anaesthetist.

Adrenaline Adrenaline has both α- and β-adrenergic stimulatory effects. The α effect results in vasoconstriction which increases coronary perfusion. Adrenaline is used primarily in the treatment of asystole, but an infusion may be used in severe hypotension.

The initial dose of adrenaline is 10 μg/kg and this should be increased ten-fold in subsequent doses. Acidosis renders adrenaline less effective. It is inactivated by sodium bicarbonate, and so a saline flush should be used first if adrenaline injection follows sodium bicarbonate.

Atropine Atropine increases the heart rate by increasing the rate of discharge from the sinoatrial node and increasing conduction through the atrioventricular node. The indication for atropine is bradycardia with a poor cardiac output despite

Table 2.4 • Drugs for the paediatric resuscitation area

Drugs	Presentation
Adrenaline	1:10 000
Atropine	600 μg/ml
Sodium bicarbonate	8.4%
Dopamine	40 mg/ml
Lignocaine	1%
Dextrose	25% + 50%
Calcium chloride	10%
Frusemide	20 mg/ml
Mannitol	10% + 20%
Antibiotics—penicillin, gentamicin, ampicillin, cefotaxime	

adequate ventilation. It can be given following adrenaline in asystole if vagal stimulation is thought to have contributed to cardiac arrest. The minimum dose is 0.1 mg.

Sodium bicarbonate Sodium bicarbonate is used for the correction of metabolic acidosis. Acidosis can be demonstrated by analysis of blood gas sample, or can be assumed to be present in a patient who has had circulatory arrest for more than a few minutes. Sodium bicarbonate is an irritant and hyperosmolar drug which contains a high concentration of sodium. It dissociates into carbon dioxide which can cause intracellular acidosis, though it will temporarily raise the intravascular pH. If the patient is being ventilated, some carbon dioxide can be removed by hyperventilation while the bicarbonate is being infused.

The drug is now used more sparingly than in the past. However, children in cardiac arrest are likely to be very acidotic from preceding respiratory or circulatory failure, and it is appropriate to use bicarbonate in paediatric CPR. The dose for children is 1 mmol/kg (1 ml/kg of 8.4 per cent bicarbonate), and it should be administered by a doctor or nurse with a syringe and not run in through a burette. Sodium bicarbonate must *not* be given in the same intravenous line as calcium as precipitation will occur. Sodium bicarbonate inactivates adrenaline and dopamine, and therefore the line must be flushed with saline if these drugs are given subsequently. Bicarbonate may not be given by the intratracheal route.

Dopamine Dopamine is indicated for the patient who has cardiac activity and output but inadequate renal perfusion despite sufficient volume replacement. At an infusion of 2–10 µg/kg/min, dopamine increases blood flow to renal and mesenteric blood vessels and will improve renal perfusion and therefore urine output in a patient with poor urine flow. In higher doses (10–20 µg/kg/min) it has an inotropic effect.

Dobutamine Dobutamine increases cardiac output by increasing cardiac contractility and heart rate. The initial dose is 10 µg/kg/min. Low dose dopamine and dobutamine at the recommended dose can be used together.

Catecholamines can produce tachycardia and ectopic cardiac beats; hence careful monitoring of the blood pressure and cardiac rhythm is necessary. As extravasation of the drug into subcutaneous tissues may cause damage, it should be given through a central line whenever possible.

Lignocaine Ventricular fibrillation is a relatively uncommon event and is usually treated with cardioversion. However, if repeated defibrillation is unsuccessful, even after a dose of adrenaline, lignocaine at a dose of 1 mg/kg may be given intravenously before a further defibrillation attempt.

Calcium Calcium is rarely used in resuscitation. It is occasionally needed for treating hyperkalaemia or hypocalcaemia. It is of no use in asystole. Calcium chloride is given at 10 mg/kg. Calcium may have serious toxic effects, particularly causing bradycardia, coronary artery spasm, and myocardial irritability. It causes severe local tissue necrosis if injected outside a vein.

Frusemide This diuretic is occasionally used following cardiopulmonary resuscitation after the patient has established cardiac output and if there is no urine production in the face of acute pulmonary oedema. The initial dose is 1 mg/kg intravenously. However, hypovolaemia or poor cardiac contractility are also causes of poor urine output and should also be addressed in patients with anuria. Following resuscitation, a urine output of 2 ml/kg/h in infants and 1 ml/kg/h in children is adequate.

Mannitol This osmotic diuretic is used when there is evidence of life-threatening raised intracranial pressure, as shown by dilating pupils, slowing pulse, and increasing blood pressure, or a decrease in level of consciousness not caused by hypoxia, hypovolaemia, etc.

Table 2.5 • Intravenous fluids for the paediatric resuscitation area

0.9% Saline
4% Dextrose and 0.18% saline
5% Dextrose
Hartmann's solution or Ringer's lactate
Colloid, e.g. Haemaccel
Plasma
5% Human albumin

Monitoring in CPR

1. ECG—leads should be attached at the periphery of the chest or on limbs so as not to obscure any X-ray appearances.

2. Core temperature—a continuously reading rectal temperature probe should be used. A low-reading thermometer is also needed for small infants who may easily become hypothermic.

3. Oxygen saturation—a pulse oximeter should be attached to a digit or foot in the case of a small infant. A saturation of over 95 per cent should be aimed for. The instrument is inaccurate when circulation is poor.

4. Non-invasive blood pressure—a blood pressure monitoring device should be recording at two-minute intervals on a limb not needed for intravenous access. Ensure that the correct sized cuff is used. The width of the cuff should be two-thirds of the length of the child's upper arm.

5. Urine output—following the resumption of effective cardiac action a urinary catheter should be inserted and all output measured.

Post-resuscitation management

- **Airway and breathing   Circulation   Cerebral management   Investigations and further treatment following CPR   Hypothermia   Transport   When to stop resuscitation**

The survivors of resuscitation vary from those, usually with a respiratory arrest only, who are apparently fully recovered to the unconscious child with multisystem failure. Again, a systematic approach is necessary to maximize the patient's outcome. Management of this stage is a paediatric and anaesthetic responsibility. Monitoring of ECG, blood pressure, and oxygen saturation should continue.

Airway and breathing

Many post-resuscitation patients will have an impaired level of consciousness or depressed gag reflex. In most cases the child should remain intubated and the decision to extubate should be made by senior paediatric or anaesthetic staff.

Adequate oxygenation is vital; an arterial blood gas sample will give information on this, pco_2, and acid–base status. Ventilation with a concentration of oxygen sufficient to keep the patient's oxygen saturation above 95 per cent, as measured on a pulse oximeter, should be continued if there are any doubts about the patient's ventilatory status.

Circulation

There is often poor cardiac output following resuscitation. This may result from both the underlying illness or injury and the damaging effects of hypoxia and ischaemia on the heart and circulation. If there is poor cardiac output, as shown by hypotension and poor peripheral perfusion, an initial bolus of 20 ml/kg of plasma or a colloid should be given and its clinical effect noted. A further 20 ml/kg may be given if the first had no useful effect and if there is no evidence of fluid overload, such as distended neck veins. At the same time a central venous pressure (CVP) line should be placed; the external jugular or femoral veins are the usual sites for cannulation. This will usually be performed in the intensive care unit but may occasionally be necessary in the A & E department. The procedure should only be undertaken by a skilled person.

The CVP is principally a measure of right ventricular function and of the effect of venous return on pre-load. The CVP is best utilized in assessing the response to a fluid challenge. The CVP of a hypovolaemic patient will change little in response to an initial fluid bolus, but the CVP of a patient who is euvolaemic, hypervolaemic, or in cardiogenic shock will have a large sustained increase with a fluid challenge. A CVP of less than 10 mmHg indicates the need for further volume replacement. Above this level, the need is probably for inotropic cardiac support and an intravenous infusion of dopamine and/or dobutamine should be started through the central line.

If it is not possible to obtain a CVP line and poor perfusion continues, inotrope infusion should be started, through a peripheral vein, at the same time as a third fluid challenge of 10 ml/kg of colloid.

Transfer should be made to intensive care where more invasive monitoring of cardiac output may be necessary to ensure optimum treatment.

A urinary catheter should be passed and all urinary output measured and charted. A rate of 2 ml/kg/h in an infant and 1 ml/kg/h in a child is evidence of reasonable renal perfusion and function.

Cerebral management

In some cases the brain will have suffered damage from hypoxia and ischaemia before and during CPR. It is important to avoid further insult during the post-resuscitation period by the following strategies.

- Ensure good oxygenation.
- avoid hypo- and hypertension.
- Keep the patient normothermic.
- Avoid hypo- and hyperglycaemia.
- Treat acid–base abnormalities.
- Help to reduce raised intracranial pressure by hyperventilation (arterial $p\text{CO}_2$ of 28–30 mmHg).
- Nurse the patient in the 30° head-up position.
- Avoid painful or unpleasant procedures, which cause surges in arterial blood pressure, without adequate pain relief.
- If there is evidence of raised intracranial pressure as shown by falling conscious level, the development of neurological signs such as sixth nerve palsy, or a slowing pulse, intravenous mannitol may be used.

Investigations and further treatment following CPR

The most important investigation is arterial blood gas sampling to determine oxygenation, ventilatory adequacy, and acid–base balance. Sodium bicarbonate may be needed if there is a pronounced metabolic acidosis and should be given initially as a slow bolus (over 5 min) of 1 mmol/kg. Blood may be taken for serum electrolyte and urea estimations, as well as for a haemoglobin and a blood film.

A blood culture should be taken, and if there is any suggestion that infection is a possible cause of the child's collapse, antibiotics should be given (see p. 35).

A chest radiograph is needed to show the position of the ET tube and any pulmonary pathology. Further investigations will depend on the underlying pathology.

Hypothermia

Sick children, especially very young ones, can become hypothermic when exposed to cold for even short periods. Try to prevent this by keeping the child covered or under an overhead heater without compromising access or observation. Monitor rectal temperature.

Transport

Once resuscitation has achieved cardiorespiratory stability, most patients will require intensive care. This may be in the receiving hospital or may require transfer to another hospital. In either circumstance patients should be transferred:

- with endotracheal intubation and ventilatory support
- with appropriately trained personnel in attendance, for example an anaesthetist
- with drugs and equipment for further resuscitation on the journey (see Tables 2.3 and 2.4).

If the patient is to be transferred to another hospital it is wise to discuss transport needs with the receiving team; some intensive care units have a mobile team who will come to transport the patient back to their unit.

When to stop resuscitation

If an initially apnoeic pulseless patient has had no detectable signs of cardiac output and no evidence of cerebral activity despite 30 minutes of CPR it is reasonable to stop resuscitation. The decision to stop CPR is taken by the team leader, but it is appropriate to ensure that all team members are in agreement.

The exception to the above is the hypothermic patient in whom resuscitation must continue until the patient has a core temperature of at least 32°C (see p. 37).

Laryngeal or tracheal obstruction management

If foreign body aspiration has been witnessed or is strongly suspected and the child is coughing forcefully, encourage him to continue trying to dislodge the obstruction himself and give oxygen in high concentration. As long as the child is able to move air there is only partial obstruction. Attempts to dislodge the foreign body should not be undertaken at this stage as this may convert the partial obstruction into a complete one. *A senior anaesthetist and ear, nose, and throat (ENT) surgeon should be urgently called to the child.* The ENT surgeon will probably remove the obstruction by direct laryngoscopy, but operative intervention may be necessary.

A lateral radiograph of the neck may reveal a radio-opaque foreign body in the upper airway or oesophagus. A child in respiratory distress should not be X-rayed but should proceed to laryngoscopy by an experienced person. If radiography is needed, an experienced doctor should accompany the child.

However, if the child is blue or there is no evidence of air movement, emergency management in the A & E department is necessary. First, remove any obvious foreign body manually or with forceps, making sure that the procedure does not traumatize the mucosa or push the foreign body further down.

Infants less than one year old should be placed prone with the head dependent over the operator's knees and five back blows given in rapid succession (Fig. 2.5). If this is not successful, the infant should be placed supine on a firm surface and given five chest thrusts. Small children aged between one and five years should be placed supine on a firm surface and given five midline abdominal thrusts in the upper abdomen.

For children over five years of age the Heimlich manoeuvre can be performed. In this, the patient's abdomen is grasped from behind and a sharp upward squeeze is given in the subdiaphragmatic area is given (Fig. 2.6). This may be accompanied by back blows. The Heimlich manoeuvre can also be performed with the patient supine.

If these manoeuvres are unsuccessful and there is still no air movement, rapid direct laryngoscopy should be attempted to see if the foreign body is removable with forceps. If it is not, then an emergency cricothyrotomy should be performed (see p. 68).

Recognition of the seriously ill child

- **Imminent respiratory failure   Signs of early circulatory failure**

As described earlier, cardiac arrest in childhood is usually secondary to respiratory or circulatory failure. Recognition of the early stages of these problems allows early management which may avert deterioration.

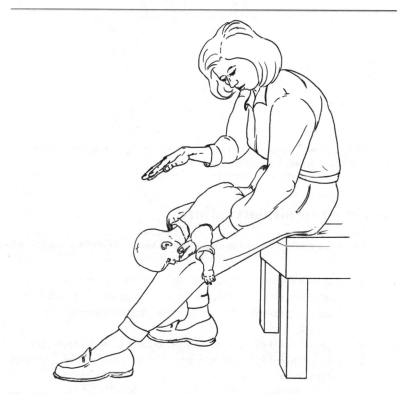

Fig 2.5 • Emergency management of upper-airway obstruction in infants and young children.

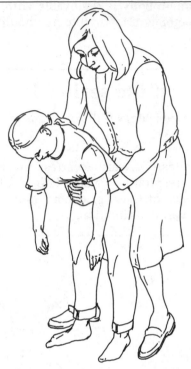

Fig. 2.6 • The Heimlich manoeuvre for upper-airway obstruction in children aged five years and over.

Imminent respiratory failure

> Box 2.1 **Signs suggestive of imminent respiratory failure**
>
> - Severe chest retraction, tachypnoea, and use of accessory muscles of respiration (these signs diminish as the patient either improves with treatment or worsens with fatigue)
> - Decreased or absent breath sounds on auscultation
> - Decreased level of consciousness or restlessness and agitation
> - Hypotonia
> - Cyanosis

Children with the signs shown in Box 2.1 require a high concentration of oxygen at 15 litres/minute by mask and specific treatment of the underlying respiratory complaint should be given. *Paediatric and anaesthetic help should be sought urgently.* If the respiratory rate is falling because the child is exhausted, artificial ventilation with oxygen via a bag and mask will be necessary until intubation can be performed, preferably by an experienced person.

Signs of early circulatory failure

Shock can develop rapidly in children because the loss of relatively small amounts of fluid may comprise a high percentage of their intravascular volume. Children have approximately 80 ml of blood per kilogram body weight. In addition, children initially compensate well for fluid loss with few physical signs until more than one-third of the circulating volume is lost. Shock then develops rapidly.

Box 2.2 **Signs of circulatory failure**

1. Rapid thready pulse (compensation for diminished stroke volume)
2. Rapid deep breathing (acidosis from peripheral ischaemia)
3. Agitation or depressed conscious level (caused by poor cerebral perfusion)
4. Skin pallor and coldness with poor capillary refill (vasoconstriction to preserve essential organs)—capillary refill after cutaneous pressure for five seconds should occur within two to three seconds; a refill time of more than five seconds is clearly abnormal
5. Hypotension—this is a late sign of circulatory failure; expected systolic blood pressure can be estimated by the formula
   blood pressure = 80 + (age in years 2)

Treatment of children in circulatory failure

Intravenous or intraosseous access must be secured immediately and 20 ml/kg of colloid or crystalloid infused as rapidly as possible.

Table 2.6 • Acceptable upper limits for physiological parameters in awake children

Age group	Respiratory rate	Pulse rate
Infant	50	160
Toddler	35	140
School age	25	120
Adolescent	20	110

Oxygen must be given and the patient reassessed; further boluses of fluid may be required.

Some specific problems

**Septicaemia   Meningococcal septicaemia   Reye's syndrome
Diabetic ketoacidosis   Haemolytic uraemic syndrome
Hypothermia   Drowning   Anaphylactic shock   Heat stroke
Supraventricular tachycardia**

The following are serious illnesses and conditions which, while not exclusive to childhood, are encountered particularly in this age group. Other life-threatening conditions which are largely confined to one organ system are described in the appropriate chapters, for example epiglottitis (p. 172) and meningitis (p. 216/220). *Urgent senior paediatric help should be sought in each instance.*

Septicaemia

There should be a high index of suspicion for the possibility of bacterial infection in children who become rapidly and seriously ill, especially those aged under two years. Unless there is clear evidence of a specific alternative diagnosis, very ill children with shock should be treated with intravenous antibiotics, as well as receiving supportive therapy. A blood culture should be taken first.

The most common bacterial pathogen is now *Neisseria meningitidis. Streptococcus pneumoniae* and *Haemophilus influenzae* are less common; the frequency of the latter has been reduced following the recent introduction of the Hib

vaccine. Infection with *Staphylococcus* spp. *Eschierichia, coli, Salmonella* spp. and *Shigella* spp. occurs less frequently. In neo-nates, Gram-negative organisms are more common and beta haemolytic streptococcus is an important pathogen. In addition to oxygen and intravenous colloid, septicaemic children should be given intravenous penicillin and a broad-spectrum antibiotic, such as gentamicin or cefotaxime, which is active against Gram-negative organisms.

Meningococcal septicaemia

Meningococcal septicaemia is the most fulminant infectious disease. The interval from the first symptom to death can be less than 12 hours. Some patients complain of a sore throat the onset of the disease; others are simply febrile and ill. The cardinal sign of meningococcal septicaemia is a purpuric rash in an ill child. At the onset, the rash is not florid and a careful search should be made for purpura in any unwell child. In about 10 per cent of patients with meningococcal septicaemia an initial blanching erythematous rash precedes a purpuric rash, and in some cases no rash occurs.

Purpura is caused by vasculitis and disseminated intravascular coagulation, both of which are the result of endotoxins produced by the organism *N. meningitidis*. Although the majority of patients who survive have no long-term sequelae, some have ischaemic skin or limb loss.

Management If meningococcal septicaemia is suspected, a blood culture and full blood count should be taken, and intravenous benzyl penicillin 50 mg/kg up to a maximum of 2 g given immediately. The antibiotics should be given over five to ten minutes, as more rapid infusion of such a high dose could cause convulsions. If the patient is showing signs of shock, intravenous colloid should be given at 20 ml/kg initially. Further boluses are usually necessary after reassessment. These patients should be urgently referred to the paediatrician and many will need transfer to an intensive care unit. A poor prognosis is associated with those who present with a low white cell count or shock. If the patient is allergic to penicillin, intravenous erythromycin or aztreonam can be given. It is common practice to give a third-generation cephalosporin as well as penicillin.

Reye's syndrome

This relatively uncommon condition is characterized by a rapidly progressive encephalopathy with hypoglycaemia and fatty changes in the liver. Some cases follow varicella or influenza infection. These children appear to improve from their first illness and then become unwell again with profuse vomiting and progressive drowsiness. Other children do not appear to have a prodromal illness. An alleged association with aspirin has led to the banning of aspirin for general use in children less than 12 years of age.

Children with Reye's syndrome present to the A & E department with vomiting, drowsiness, convulsions, or coma. The liver is palpably enlarged and firm. The blood sugar is very low, and liver enzymes and serum ammonia are raised.

Although the condition is relatively uncommon, a high index of suspicion should be maintained for Reye's syndrome in patients presenting with profuse vomiting, neurological changes, or hypoglycaemia. Patients can make a good recovery if the disease is recognized early and vigorous treatment instituted rapidly.

The mainstays of treatment are management of the hypoglycaemia and the raised intracranial pressure. For the latter the patient needs to be transferred to a paediatric intensive care unit for intracranial pressure monitoring and treatment of raised intracranial pressure. While awaiting transfer the patient should be kept in a head-up position and fluids should be restricted. If there is continuing deterioration, intubation and ventilation should be instituted and intravenous mannitol given.

Diabetic ketoacidosis

Ketoacidosis is found at presentation in 30 per cent of newly diagnosed diabetic children. Patients may present at A & E departments with

- a history of poluria and polydipsia
- weight loss and dehydration
- abdominal pain and vomiting (sometimes misdiagnosed as appendicitis)
- rapid respiration (sometimes misdiagnosed as pneumonia or asthma)
- coma

On examination children with diabetic ketoacidosis are dehydrated and acidotic with rapid deep breathing. The conscious level may be decreased, and in severe cases there may be signs of shock with a rapid pulse and cold extremities.

The initial treatment is to correct dehydration. Intravenous access should be secured and 10–20 ml/kg of normal saline infused over the first hour unless shock requires a more rapid infusion of colloid. Blood should be taken for measurement of glucose, urea, and electrolytes, and an arterial blood sample for acid–base status. The paediatric team should have taken over the patient's care at this stage and will probably infuse insulin at the rate of 0.1 unit/kg/h once the blood sugar result is known as well as starting potassium replacement. Despite metabolic acidosis, intravenous sodium bicarbonate is rarely indicated, as replacement of fluid and electrolytes usually corrects the acidosis. The patient's neurological status should be carefully monitored as a few diabetic children (even those who are mildly affected) may develop fatal cerebral oedema.

Haemolytic uraemic syndrome

This relatively uncommon condition affects approximately 150 children each year in the UK. It comprises a micro-angiopathic haemolytic anaemia, thrombocytopenia, and acute renal failure. Most cases follow a diarrhoeal illness (often with bloody stools) caused by *E. coli* or *Shigella* spp. and it is thought that a toxin produced by these organisms initiates the disease.

The patient presents to the A & E department with diarrhoea, pallor, or anuria. On examination the patient is unwell and pale, some petechiae may be seen, and some patients are hypertensive. The diagnosis is suspected on examination of a blood film which will show anaemia, red blood cell fragmentation, and thrombocytopenia. The blood urea level will be raised. It is important to restrict fluids in these patients as their renal function is compromised. They usually need dialysis.

Hypothermia

Profound hypothermia rarely occurs in children with the exception of the near-drowned patient. Mild hypothermia (temperature usually over 32°C) occurs in small babies, often in association with an infection. It may also occur in those handicapped children who are undernourished and immobile.

In all cases of mild hypothermia, the patient should be warmed by wrapping with warmed blankets in a warm draught-free room, or with an overhead radiant heater in the case of infants. Infants warmed by radiant heat may be covered in 'bubble' polythene to insulate and reduce convection losses while allowing radiant heat to penetrate the covering. Continuous rectal temperature and ECG monitoring are needed. Admission, screening, and treatment for infection will be necessary.

Drowning

Most drowning incidents in this country are in freshwater canals and lakes, domestic swimming pools, and, in infants, the domestic bath.

Two main problems in the drowned patient are hypoxia and hypothermia. In 15 per cent of cases hypoxia is caused by laryngospasm which prevents water from entering the lung—'dry drowning'. In the other 85 per cent flooding of fresh water into the lungs causes alveolar damage and pulmonary oedema.

Hypothermia leads to bradycardia and asystole with circulatory shutdown and the development of acidosis.

However, hypothermia may have a minor protective effect in some cases of near-drowning. In addition, there is a small protective effect from the 'dive reflex'. This is a reflex, weak in humans, which, following sudden immersion in cold water, causes peripheral and splanchnic vasoconstriction shunting blood primarily to the brain and heart and giving those organs perfusion for a few more minutes.

Haemolysis or electrolyte problems caused by the inhalation or ingestion of large amounts of water are unusual.

Management of the near-drowned patient All victims must be hospitalized for at least 24 hours even if they seem well, as late respiratory sequelae may occur. It is important to find out if the patient has a history of epilepsy, diabetes, or drug abuse problems which may have precipitated the near-drowning episode and also require treatment.

For those patients who are admitted in asystole or respiratory arrest, cardiopulmonary resuscitation should be carried out with cervical spine protection. After resuscitation, the patient must be examined for additional trauma, such as a head or neck injury which may have occurred before or during the near-drowning episode.

The patient's core temperature should be measured using a low-reading thermometer which can read down to 15 °C. Warming procedures should be instituted. If the core temperature is above 30°C, external re-warming with blankets or radiant heaters is usually sufficient. For a core temperature below 30 °C, active core warming in addition to warmed blankets or radiant heaters is necessary. Core warming can be carried out by

- gastric and rectal or urinary bladder lavage with saline warmed to 40 °C
- the use of warmed humidified inspired gases via a ventilator
- warmed intravenous fluids (40 °C)
- peritoneal lavage with saline at 40 °C.

Extra-corporeal blood warming may be available in a few centres but is unlikely to be easily applicable in most hospitals.

Resuscitation should be continued in the hypothermic patient until the patient's core temperature has been at or near normal for 15 minutes. Occasional cases have been recorded where complete recovery has resulted despite cardiac arrest due to submersion in water for periods exceeding one hour.

Patients recovering from near-drowning may develop ventricular fibrillation. This is best treated with DC shock, and is often refractory to the use of lignocaine. As the patient warms up, vasodilatation may cause relative hypovolaemia, requiring circulatory support with crystalloid or colloid.

Whether or not resuscitation has been required, the near-drowned patient should be given oxygen. A chest radiograph should be taken and the patient should have continuous ECG monitoring.

Blood should be taken for arterial blood gas, urea, electrolytes, and glucose estimations; the blood gas results should be corrected for the patient's temperature if he is still hypothermic. Patients with biochemical or radiographic abnormalities or respiratory symptoms or signs should be considered for admission to an intensive care unit as 'secondary drowning' is very likely.

Anaphylactic shock

This is a severe and occasionally life-threatening generalized allergic reaction. The main causes are

- injection of drugs, e.g. penicillin
- injection of foreign proteins, e.g. horse serum blood products
- bee, wasp, and hornet stings
- hyposensitization injections—this treatment is now virtually abandoned for hay fever because of the risk of fatal anaphylactic reaction
- X-ray contrast injections
- foods, especially peanuts

Anaphylactic shock occurs rapidly within minutes of the cause. The condition usually starts with urticaria and angioneurotic oedema (swelling of the face, eyelids, and lips). The patient may have sneezing and wheezing, leading to stridor, shock, collapse, and death. Vomiting, abdominal pain, and loose stools sometimes occur, especially when the cause has been an ingested allergen.

Management of anaphylactic shock

1. The first essential is to ensure a patent airway and to give oxygen. *Anaesthetic help should be urgently sought.* If there is obstruction of the airway, intubation, or if this is impossible, cricothyrotomy is necessary.

2. Intramuscular adrenalin should be given at a dose of 0.1 ml/ kg of 1:10 000 or 0.01 ml/kg of 1:1,000 adrenalin. If the patient has poor peripheral circulation, intravenous adrenaline is necessary but must be given with extreme caution. If venous access is difficult and the patient is intubated, the adrenaline may be given down the endotracheal tube; otherwise an intramuscular dose should be given or the intraosseous or femoral vein route should be tried (see p. 68). If there is a poor response, repeated doses of adrenaline should be given every 10 minutes.

3. General cardiorespiratory support will also be necessary with intravenous colloid and ventilation with oxygen. Nebulized salbutamol may be helpful for bronchospasm.

4. Intravenous steroids (hydrocortisone 2 mg/kg) and antihistamines (e.g. chlorpheniramime 2–10 mg) can be given, but their effect, if any, is delayed.

Heat stroke

Heat stroke occurs occasionally in infants who are too warmly wrapped during a febrile illness. It may occur if children are left unattended in a closed car in direct sunlight.

There is a suggestion that overheating is associated with the sudden infant death syndrome (see p. 259) and with the uncommon haemorrhagic encephalopathy syndrome which show similar pathological changes to heat stroke.

The core temperature is usually above 41°C in infants with heat stroke. The infant usually has circulatory collapse, may convulse, and may have diarrhoea and vomiting.

The infant must be cooled rapidly. This is usually quickly achieved by wetting and fanning the exposed skin. Rectal paracetamol should be given.

Supportive care with oxygen, ventilation, and intravenous colloid is often necessary. The paediatrician should be called urgently. Infection is usually associated with the hyperthermia and should be treated appropriately (see p. 34).

The infant will usually require intensive care as brain swelling and clotting disorders often develop.

Supraventricular tachycardia

Most babies with supraventricular tachycardia present with poor feeding and tachypnoea.

The diagnosis is suggested by noting the extremely rapid heart rate. Occasionally it can be difficult to distinguish clinically between supraventricular tachycardia and sinus tachycardia in an ill infant. A rate of 250 beats/minute is a supraventricular tachycardia, but rates between 200 and 220 beats/minute may be a sinus tachycardia in an infant. An ECG should clarify this and allow the heart rate to be measured accurately.

The baby should be given oxygen in high concentration by mask, and urgent paediatric help should be sought.

A good treatment for supraventricular tachycardia in early infancy is to elicit the 'diving reflex' which produces an increase in vagal tone, slows atrioventricular conduction, and interrupts the tachycardia. The baby should be attached to an electrocardiographic monitor, wrapped in a towel, and his whole face immersed in iced water for about five seconds.

There is no need to obstruct the mouth or nostrils as the baby will be temporarily apnoeic. The tachycardia will usually stop immediately, but may be delayed for a few seconds. There may be bradycardia for a short while until normal sinus rhythm returns. If the infant is in shock he should receive a synchronized DC shock of an initial dose of 0.5 J/kg. Adenosine is a safe antiarrhythmic drug which can be used as an alternative to DC shock. Urgent paediatric advice should be sought and a paediatric cardiologist contacted.

Note: Verapamil is no longer considered safe to give to the paediatric age group and especially to infants; although the drug is effective in stopping supraventricular tachycardia it has caused asystole in a number of patients.

Further reading

1. Advanced Life Support Group (1993). *Advanced paediatric life support—the practical approach*. BMJ, London.
2. Levin, D. C. and Morris, F. C. (ed.) (1990). *Essentials of paediatric intensive care*. Quality Medical Publications, St Louis, MO.

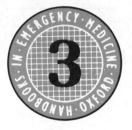

Major trauma

Key points in major trauma

1   The first priority is to ensure a patent airway and adequate ventilation with 100 per cent oxygen.

2   Intravenous access should be obtained with two large cannulae. A child can sustain a relatively large blood loss with initial compensation. Shock then develops rapidly.

3   A detailed history of the accident will help to anticipate the nature and severity of injuries.

4   Suspect internal chest injury if there is continuing hypoxia in a ventilated patient. Children may have severe chest cavity injuries despite intact ribs.

5   Abdominal and pelvic injury are particularly common and difficult to detect in children. Repeated abdominal examination, CT and ultrasound scans, and peritoneal lavage will all help in assessment. The patient with suspected abdominal injury who cannot be made haemodynamically stable with ventilation and transfusion must go for urgent surgical exploration. Exact pre-operative diagnosis is unnecessary.

6   The management of head injuries should focus on prevention of secondary damage from hypoxia, hypotension, and raised intracranial pressure.

Introduction

Accidents cause about 700 deaths a year in children in England and Wales. Fifty-five per cent of these are the result of road traffic accidents and 29 per cent are due to accidents in the home. The main cause of death is head injury (with brain swelling).

Most road traffic accident deaths in children occur in pedestrians (250 per year); about 70 deaths per year occur in cyclists.

Most home fatalities are due to asphyxia from house fires, and about 60 deaths a year are the result of falls in the home.

Many of these deaths are avoidable. Firstly, accidents should be prevented: children should be well supervised and dangerous situations avoided; the urban environment and vehicles should be designed with safety in mind; homes should be equipped with smoke alarms; safety glass should be installed in doors and windows, and child-proof tops should be used for drugs and household products. Secondly, the injuries caused by accidents can be minimized by the use of safety devices such as seat belts and cycle helmets. Thirdly, prompt and effective treatment of the injured child will improve the outcome.

The early management of the multiply injured child is crucial, not only for the immediate problems but also for long-term rehabilitation. Untreated hypoxia and shock will have adverse short- and long-term effects. The first hours after the accident are the most important in this regard. A major difficulty is how to assess the severity of the child's injuries quickly. Trauma scores have been used in the assessment of adults with major trauma for some time; however, the disadvantage of a trauma score is that it can give a falsely benign result if calculated very soon after the injury. Additional difficulties encountered with children are unfamiliarity with the score because of infrequent use and a lack of verification of its widespread applicability in the UK. Table 3.1 shows a paediatric trauma score adapted from the Advanced Trauma Life Support (ATLS) Course. A score of less than 8 is used in the USA to indicate to on-scene paramedics that the child should be admitted to a Paediatric Trauma Unit.

When faced with a child with severe or multiple trauma call

Table 3.1 • Paediatric trauma score

Score	+2	+1	-1
Size	> 20 kg	1–20 kg	< 10 kg
Airway	Normal	Oral or nasal airway	Intubated
Systolic BP	> 90 mmHg	90–50 mmHg	< 50 mmHg
Level of consciousness	Fully awake	Drowsy	Unconscious
Open wound	None	Minor	Major/penetrating
Fractures	None	Minor	Open or multiple

for senior help immediately. Many hospitals have a 'trauma team' consisting of an anaesthetist and one or more surgeons. The surgeon will take over the patient's care and call in specialist surgeons for neuro-surgery, orthopaedics, etc. as appropriate and if they are available.

The management of major trauma has been improved by training doctors on the ATLS Course and the Advanced Paediatric Life Support Course. The approved method is to adopt the following scheme of management:

• primary survey
• resuscitation
• secondary survey (total evaluation of the patient)

• definitive care.

In the primary survey the ABCDE of priorities is followed:

• **A**irway with cervical spine control
• **B**reathing
• **C**irculation with haemorrhage control
• **D**isability—brief neurological evaluation
• **E**xposure—completely undress the patient

If the above schemes are followed, the resuscitation will take place in an ordered and rational way.

There are several differences between children and adults that have implications for treatment. Children are smaller than adults, and therefore they are a smaller target if hit by a vehicle. The energy of impact is dissipated over a smaller mass so that a greater force is applied to a small area; thus more severe injuries are likely to be caused. Children have less body fat, less elastic connective tissue, and closer proximity of multiple organs than adults. Thus there is a high frequency of multiple organ injury. The skeleton of the child is incompletely calci-fied and has many active growth centres. A child's bones often bend rather than break, and so there may be significant organ damage without overlying bony fracture; for example in the chest the ribs may be intact but there cold be underlying pul-monary contusion, haemorrhage, or pneumothorax.

The ratio of the child's body surface to body volume is high-est at birth and decreases during infancy and childhood. This relatively large surface area increases heat loss. It is important to ensure that any fluids or gases that are given are warmed, if time permits, and that the child is covered with a blanket and/or an overhead heater is used. An additional difficulty is that frightened children may not cooperate. Reassurance and, if possible, a parent's presence are very important.

Primary survey and resuscitation

- **Airway with cervical spine control   Breathing Life-threatening problems with respiration   Circulation with haemorrhage control   Disability   Other procedures carried out during the primary survey and resuscitation**

During the primary survey, life-threatening conditions are identified and the appropriate resuscitative measures are taken as soon as a problem is found.

Airway with cervical spine control

The patency of the airway should be assessed by **looking** for chest movements, **listening** for breath sounds, and **feeling** for exhaled breath. If there is no evidence of air movement, an air-way-opening manoeuvre should be performed. This should be a jaw-thrust manoeuvre as the chin-lift–head-tilt manoeuvre is contraindicated in trauma. If there is still no air movement, ventilation with a self-inflating bag and mask should be com-menced. If there is difficulty in ventilating the patient, airway obstruction should be suspected. This is first dealt with by attempting another airway-opening manoeuvre. If this is unsuccessful, the airway should be inspected and cleared if possible by suction. The patient may be intubated or, if this is not possible because of upper-airway injury, a cricothyrotomy may be indicated (see p. 68).

Early intubation should be undertaken in any patient with facial or upper-airway burns as later oedema may make airway control difficult. Equally, consideration should be given to early intubation in patients with significant facial injuries for the same reason. Planned intubation should always be carried out by an anaesthetist using rapid induction anaesthesia. Non-anaesthetists should only intubate patients in an emergency. The airway management sequence is summarized in Box 3.1.

Box 3.1 **Airway management sequence**

- Jaw thrust
- Suction/removal of foreign body
- Oral/pharyngeal airways
- Endotracheal intubation
- Cricothyrotomy or surgical airway

In any patient with significant trauma, the cervical spine should be presumed to be damaged until proved intact. Children can have spinal cord injury without radiographic abnormality (SCIWORA syndrome). The head and neck should be immobilized initially by in-line manual stabilization. When the patient's condition permits, use a hard collar properly sized and applied with additional sandbags taped to each side of the head. Uncooperative patients should simply have a hard collar applied because too rigid immobilization of the head in struggling patients may increase neck movement. Immobilizing manoeuvres may only be discontinued when both radiographs are normal and the neurological examination has been demonstrated to be completely normal. This may not be for some days if the patient is paralysed for ventilation.

Breathing

Once the airway has been assessed and secured if necessary and the cervical spine controlled, breathing should be assessed. High flow oxygen should be given immediately. The adequacy of respiration is assessed from looking at the work of breathing, the effectiveness of breathing, and the effects of inadequate breathing on other organ systems. These observations are summarized in Box 3.2.

Box 3.2 Assessment of respiration

- Work of breathing
  Respiratory rate
  Recession
  Inspiratory or expiratory noises
  Accessory muscle use
- Effectiveness of breathing
  Auscultation of the chest
  Chest expansion
  Pulse oximetry
- Effects of inadequate respiration
  Bradycardia or tachycardia
  Pallor or cyanosis
  Agitation or drowsiness

If the breathing is inadequate, ventilation must be started. This is initially by bag and mask, but usually intubation is necessary if ventilatory support is required. The indications for intubation and ventilation are summarized in Box 3.3.

Box 3.3 Indications for intubation

- Apnoea
- Moderate or severe respiratory distress or hypoxia
- Obstruction of the upper airway
- Absent gag reflex—intubation protects the lower airway from aspiration of vomit
- Severe head injury—hyperventilation may be needed to lower intracranial pressure, and control of ventilation to prevent hypoxia and hypercapnia is vital
- Severe facial or oral injuries, e.g. burns
- Flail chest
- Shock

Life-threatening problems with respiration

Tension pneumothorax In this life-threatening emergency, air accumulates in the pleural space, pushing the mediastinum across the chest. The venous return is compromised, cardiac output is reduced, and the patient is severely hypoxic. The diagnosis of a tension pneumothorax is clinical. There is no time to take a radiograph. The physical signs of tension pneumothorax are hypoxia, sometimes associated with shock. There is decreased air entry and hyper-resonance to percussion on the side of the pneumothorax. In severe cases the trachea will be deviated away from the side of the pneumothorax.

Treatment is high flow oxygen through a reservoir mask and needle thoracocentesis (see p. 67). A chest drain should be inserted subsequently to prevent recurrence.

Haemopneumothorax Damage to the lung and/or blood vessels causes both air and blood to accumulate in the pleural space.

A child with a haemopneumothorax will be hypoxic and shocked. There will be decreased chest movement, decreased air entry, and decreased resonance to percussion on the side of the haemopneumothorax.

Treatment is with high flow oxygen and ventilatory support. Intravenous access should be established and volume replacement commenced. A large chest drain should be inserted urgently.

Open pneumothorax This is an unusual injury in a child as it is usually associated with a stabbing incident. There is a penetrating wound in the chest wall with an associated pneumothorax. The wound may not be obvious as it may be on the patient's back. In a child with an open pneumothorax air will be heard sucking and blowing through the wound, and the other signs of pneumothorax will be found.

Treatment is with high flow oxygen and ventilatory support. The wound should be occluded on three sides only in order to allow air to escape and a chest drain should be inserted urgently.

Flail chest Flail chest is caused by multiple rib fractures making one section of the chest wall 'detached' from the rest of the rib cage. Because of children's flexible rib cages, this injury is uncommon, but when it does occur it indicates extremely severe chest compression. The child with a flail chest is hypoxic and rib crepitus may be felt. The child should be treated with oxygen and ventilatory support together with pain relief.

Cardiac tamponade This is also an unusual injury in children but can occur after both penetrating and blunt injury. Blood accumulates in the pericardial sac, compressing the heart and reducing stroke volume. A child with pericardial tamponade has muffled heart sounds and distended neck veins (these may not be apparent if there is also significant hypovolaemia), and is significantly shocked.

Treatment is with high flow oxygen and ventilatory support. Intravenous access should be established and volume replacement commenced. Needle pericardiocentesis should be performed (see p. 67).

Box 3.4 summarizes causes of inadequate ventilation after intubation.

Box 3.4 Causes of inadequate ventilation after intubation

- ET tube in wrong place
- Obstruction of the endotracheal tube by blood or vomit
- Pneumothorax
- Haemothorax
- Lung contusion
- Flail segment

Circulation with haemorrhage control

Control obvious exsanguinating haemorrhage by pressure. The circulation is assessed by noting the heart rate, systolic blood pressure, and capillary refill time as described in Chapter 2. In addition, skin colour and temperature, respiratory rate, and mental status indicate the end-organ effects of circulatory status. Table 3.2 shows the normal physiological parameters in childhood. Table 3.3 gives a broad indication of systemic responses to blood loss in children.

Children who have received a major injury require urgent establishment of vascular access. Two relatively large intravenous cannulae are mandatory. The initial approach should

Table 3.2 • Physiological parameters in childhood

rate	Pulse rate	Systolic BP (mmHg)	Respiratory (breaths/min)
Infants	< 160	80	40
Pre-school	< 140	90	30
School-child	< 120	100	25

Weight = 2 age (yr) + 8 kg
Blood volume approximately 80 ml/kg
Blood pressure systolic 80 mmHg + 2 age (yr)
Urine output   2 ml/kg/h in infants
                      1 ml/kg/h over 2 years of age

Table 3.3 • Systemic responses to blood loss in children

	Early (< 25% blood volume loss)	Pre-hypotensive (25% blood volume loss)	Hypotensive (40% blood volume loss)
Cardiac	Increased heart rate	Increased heart rate Weak pulse volume	Frank hypotension Tachycardia to bradycardia
CNS	Lethargic Irritable Confused Argumentative	Decrease in level of consciousness, Dulled response to pain	Unconscious
Skin	Cool, clammy	Cyanotic Decreased capillary refill Cold extremities	Pale Cold Very slow capillary refill
Kidneys	Decreased urinary output Increased specific gravity	Increased blood urea	No urinary output

be to peripheral veins, usually in the antecubital fossae. If this is not possible, other routes must be used. The external jugular vein or femoral vein can be cannulated, but intraosseous infusion is a safe and rapid technique which should be used in the emergency situation if percutaneous cannulation is impossible. However, care should be taken not to insert an intraosseous needle into a fractured limb or into a limb distal to a fracture, for example the tibia where there is a possible pelvic fracture. Central venous cannulation is hazardous in small children and should not be attempted by the inexperienced.

The initial fluid bolus should be 20 ml/kg. This will constitute a quarter of the child's circulating volume. After infusion of 20 ml/kg the circulation should be reassessed. If there has been no improvement, a further bolus of 20 ml/kg should be given. There remains considerable controversy over the best choice of fluid therapy for the shocked patient. The choices lie between crystalloid (normal saline, Ringer's lactate, Hartman's solution) or colloid (4.5% human albumin, artificial colloids such as Gelofusine or Haemaccel). The advantages of crystalloids are that the fluids are rapidly available and produce no abnormal reactions. However, crystalloid is rapidly distributed throughout the extracellular space and therefore is less effective in maintaining blood volume. Colloid infusions are more effective in maintaining blood volume but there is a low risk of anaphylactic reactions. Our practice is to start with colloid in clearly shocked patients. In mildly shocked patients we start with crystalloid and change to colloid if a second 20 ml bolus is required.

In the hypovolaemic patient, if a third bolus of fluid is required it should be warm fresh blood. If a third bolus is required, ongoing concealed haemorrhage is highly likely. If no obvious site of haemorrhage exists and there is no significant respiratory embarrassment, the probable site of blood loss is the abdomen or pelvis. The abdomen should be assessed urgently to establish whether early operative intervention is necessary. It should be inspected for bruising, lacerations, and penetrating wounds, and gently palpated. If the circulation cannot be controlled after the three boluses of fluid referred to above, rapid surgical intervention is necessary.

The management of hypovolaemic shock after trauma is summarized in Box 3.5.

Box 3.5 Management of hypovolaemic shock

Crystalloid (20 ml/kg)
↓
Colloid (20 ml/kg)
↓
Blood (20 ml/kg)
↓
Urgent surgical opinion

Full cross-matching of blood takes an hour. Type-specific blood can be available in 10–15 minutes and O negative blood should be available immediately.

Disability

The assessment of the nervous system during the primary survey consists of a brief neurological examination to establish conscious level and assessment of the pupil size and reactivity. The conscious level is determined by placing the child in once of the following four categories:

A Alert
V Response to **V**oice
P Response to **P**ain
U Unresponsive

Any inequality or lack of reactivity of the pupils in association with a poor conscious level should initially lead to a reassessment of airway, breathing, and circulation, as hypoxia or ischaemia may be the cause of these neurological signs. However, if the airway is patent, breathing is adequate, and the circulation is stable, these neurological signs suggest significant head injury and a neurosurgeon should be contacted immediately. Consideration should also be given to elective intubation and ventilation (see p. 17).

Other procedures carried out during the primary survey and resuscitation

History taking The history of the incident should be sought from the child, relatives, witnesses, and ambulance personnel. Details are required about the accident itself and also the child's past medical history, including allergies, immunization status, and the time of the last meal. If the patient was injured in a road traffic accident, the following are important points to elicit in the history: car occupancy, cyclist, or pedestrian; restraints used; thrown from vehicle; speed of impact; other victims' injuries. After a fall, the height of the fall and the landing surface are important data.

Investigations At the same time that intravenous access is obtained, blood should be taken for full blood count, base-line biochemistry, and group and cross-matching.

All seriously injured children must have radiographs taken of the lateral cervical spine, chest, and pelvis. The chest radiograph should be scrutinized for a pneumothorax, opacities indicating blood, and a widened mediastinum which suggest a tamponaded great vessel rupture. The pelvic radiograph is examined for signs of pelvic fracture which suggests very severe pelvic soft tissue injury and may be a site of significant blood loss. The cervical spine radiograph is examined for integrity of the bony spine. Other radiographs will be indicated by clinical examination.

Pain relief Analgesia should be administered to any patient in pain unless there is a very strong contraindication. Morphine is the drug of choice and should be given intravenously in a dose of 0.1 mg/kg.

Other procedures A nasogastric tube should be passed to decompress the stomach. The orogastric route should be used if there is a suspicion of base-of-skull fracture. Urinary catheterization should be performed only if continuous accurate output measurement is required. Particular care must be taken in catheterizing small boys as there is a risk of causing urethral stricture.

Secondary Survey

- **Examination of the head   Examination of the neck Examination of the chest   Examination of the abdomen Examination of the pelvis and spine   Examination of the extremities   Investigations**

The secondary survey is started after the primary survey has been completed and the patient has been stabilized. Occasionally, the primary survey is not completed within the A & E department if the patient has to go to theatre for operative intervention before haemorrhage can be controlled.

Vital signs and neurological status should be reassessed continually throughout the secondary survey. Any deterioration in these parameters should lead to an immediate return to the beginning of the primary survey.

The child should be thoroughly examined from head to toe

both front and back. A systematic approach ensures that no area of the body is left out.

Examination of the head

- Inspect the head and face for bruising, haemorrhage, laceration, deformity, and CSF leak from the nose or ears.
- Palpate the skull and face bones for deformity, lacerations, tenderness, or depressions.
- Examine the eyes and ears.
- Inspect the mouth and palpate the teeth for looseness.
- Perform a neurological examination including Glasgow coma scale, pupillary reflexes, eye movements, motor reflexes, tone, and power.

Examination of the neck

If the hard collar is removed an assistant should maintain in-line stabilization of the cervical spine until it is replaced.

- Inspect the front and back of the neck for bruising and swelling.
- Palpate the spine for tenderness, swelling, or deformity.
- Palpate for surgical emphysema.

Examination of the chest

- Inspect for bruising, deformity, abnormal movement, and lacerations.
- Inspect the neck veins for engorgement.
- Feel for tracheal deviation.
- Feel for tenderness or crepitus.
- Percuss both sides of the chest.
- Listen for breath sounds throughout the chest.
- Listen for character of heart sounds.

Examination of the abdomen

- Inspect for bruising, swellings and lacerations.
- Palpate for tenderness, masses or rigidity.
- Auscultate for bowel sounds.

Vaginal and rectal examination should be performed only by the surgeon as these examinations are distressing to children.

Examination of the pelvis and spine

The spinal examination can only be carried out after the child has been appropriately log-rolled.

- Inspect for lacerations, bruising, and deformity.
- Palpate for tenderness, swelling, and deformity.
- Inspect the perineum and external urethral meatus.
- Press over the anterior iliac crest for pain suggesting fractured pelvis.
- Assess motory and sensory function.
- Test the urine for blood.

Examination of the extremities

- Observe the limbs for deformity, bruising, or swelling.
- Palpate for tenderness (do not elicit crepitus or abnormal movement intentionally).
- Assess pulses and capillary return.
- Assess peripheral sensation to touch and prick.

Investigations

A full blood count, urea and electrolytes, and blood for group and cross-matching will have already been drawn during the primary survey. An amylase estimation should also be requested, and repeated monitoring of these investigations may be appropriate in some patients. Arterial blood gas determinations are necessary to monitor oxygen and acid–base status.

Serious injuries discovered after resuscitation

- **Chest   Abdominal injuries   Head injuries   Spinal injuries   Limb injuries   Crush injuries   Amputations Transfer of injured patients   Emergency practical procedures   Continuous assessment**

Chest

Pulmonary contusion This condition is often not identified until several hours after the injury. It is identified clinically by hypoxia requiring high flow oxygen, and on the chest radiograph as increasing radio-opacity.

Rupture of bronchus or trachea A continuous air leak after a pneumothorax has been drained suggests airway rupture. These patients should be referred to the cardiothoracic surgeon.

Disruption of the great vessels This injury is usually fatal at the site of the accident. A patient who has survived has a tamponaded tear. The diagnosis is suspected when a widened mediastinum is seen on the chest radiograph, but the patient may also be shocked and have poor peripheral pulses. Rapid cardiothoracic help is required.

Ruptured diaphragm This may occur after a blunt injury to the abdomen. The child will be hypoxic because of pulmonary compression. A chest radiograph may show bowel shadowing or an abnormal position of the nasogastric tube, indicating the presence of abdominal contents in the chest. The patient must be referred to the cardiothoracic surgeon.

Simple pneumothorax A small self-limiting pneumothorax may be seen on a chest radiograph. This may be accompanied by the presence of hyper-resonance on percussion of the chest. A chest drain should be inserted. If the patient requires ventilation for other reasons, the chest drain must be inserted urgently because in the ventilated patient a simple pneumothorax is converted to a tension pneumothorax.

Abdominal injuries

A few patients will require surgical intervention during the primary survey as part of haemorrhage control and will already have left the A & E department's care and remain under the care of the surgeons. However, most children with significant abdominal injuries do not require immediate life-saving surgery if their circulation has been stabilized.

Abdominal injury is common in major trauma in childhood as the abdomen is proportionately larger in children than in adults. Damage to solid organs such as the spleen, liver, or kidneys is common. Rupture of the bowel is less common, but hidden pelvic bleeding needs consideration.

Once the patient is stable the abdomen should be inspected for bruising, lacerations, and penetrating wounds. However, serious intra-abdominal and pelvic injury can occur without external signs, and so the presence of any visible bruising is highly suggestive. The external urethral meatus should be examined for the presence of blood. The child's abdomen should be palpated gently to reveal any areas of tenderness or rigidity. Repeated abdominal examinations form an important part of the assessment of the abdominally injured child. Internal examination should be limited to those performed by the surgeon who will take over the patient's management.

As mentioned before, gastric drainage is helpful in assessing the abdomen as acute gastric dilatation is common in injured children and may obscure important abdominal signs. Urinary catheterization should only be performed if the child cannot pass urine spontaneously or if there is a need for continuous accurate output measurement. If there are signs of urethral or bladder damage, as shown by pain or blood at the urethral meatus, an attempt at catheterization should be made by the appropriate surgeon. The catheter should be silastic and as small as possible to reduce the risk of formation of a urethral stricture.

Investigations for abdominal and pelvic injury The chest radiograph and pelvic radiograph taken during the primary survey should be re-examined, but normality does not exclude abdominal or pelvic injury. A plain abdominal radiograph may be helpful to look for the presence of free gas and the distribution of abdominal gas. Ultrasound is often readily available and can give early information on the presence of free fluid in the abdomen or pelvis, but it does not distinguish between types of fluid.

A CT scan with intravenous and intragastric contrast is the radiological investigation of choice in abdominally injured children. It will show the presence and site of a solid organ rupture, the presence or absence of two functioning kidneys, free intraperitoneal contrast from a perforated viscus, and free intraperitoneal contrast from a ruptured bladder.

Diagnostic peritoneal lavage is rarely used in children as non-operative management is now the treatment of choice for solid organ damage. Occasionally, diagnostic peritoneal lavage is necessary, for example if the child is to undergo emergency neurosurgical intervention and CT scanning of the abdomen is

not possible. It is important to remember that
fluid has been introduced, the peritoneum is irrit:
48 hours, thus reducing the accuracy of repeate(
The lavage is considered positive if the red cell count is over
100 000/mm³, the white cell count is over 500/mm³, or enteric
contents or bacteria are seen.

Management of the abdominal or pelvic injury

It has been shown over the last few years that haemorrhage
resulting from solid organ damage in children is often self-
limiting. Morbidity and mortality are reduced by a conserva-
tive approach in suitable children.

For non-operative management to be successful, the following are necessary.

1. Adequate observation and frequent monitoring: this usually
   means that the patient must be in a centre experienced in
   managing children's injuries.
2. Precise fluid management.
3. The immediate availability of a surgeon trained to operate
   on children with abdominal injuries.

Some children will always require operative intervention,
and these include those with penetrating abdominal injuries
and those with definite signs of bowel perforation. Children
whose circulation is not stable, as described in the primary
survey section, also require urgent operative intervention. If a
non-functioning kidney is demonstrated on contrast studies,
immediate exploration is necessary to see if it can be saved.

Therefore it is clearly important that children who have any
signs of possible abdominal or pelvic injury are assessed by a
paediatrically trained surgeon as early as possible. Boxes 3.5
and 3.6 show indications for surgical referral.

Head injuries

Head injury is the most common cause of death in injured
children. The damage to the brain after an accident can be
primary, as a direct result of the trauma, or secondary to other
injury factors, particularly hypoxia, hypotension, and raised
intracranial pressure.

Primary damage can be caused by direct contact between
the surface of the brain and the skull as the brain moves

Box 3.5 **Indications for surgical referral**

- External wounds or bruising to the abdomen
- Abdominal distension after nasogastric tube deflation
- Unexplained hypotension or evidence of haemorrhage
- Abdominal tenderness or guarding
- Rectal bleeding
- Lower rib fractures
- Stab wounds—examine (do not probe); if the wound is deeper than the skin the patient needs referral for a surgical opinion

Box 3.6 **Indication for referral to the genitourinary surgeon**

- Inability to pass a urethral catheter
- Urethral bleeding or bruising
- Macroscopic haematuria
- Fractured pelvis
- Abnormal intravenous pyelogram or CT scan

within its bony shell. There are also shearing forces as the brain moves and twists that damage both neurones and blood vessels.

The aim of emergency care is to prevent and treat the secondary problems in order to minimize brain damage.

Hypoxia results from airway obstruction, thoracic injuries, or inadequate ventilation caused by loss of respiratory drive secondary to brain damage. Ischaemia is caused by poor cerebral perfusion secondary to raised intracranial pressure or secondary to hypotension caused by blood loss or other causes of traumatic shock. The combination of poor systolic pressure and increasing intracranial pressure leads to a dramatic fall in cerebral perfusion pressure, causing increasing cerebral oedema and neuronal loss.

The direct effects of bleeding inside the skull include extradural and subdural haematomas. These need to be identified and drained. However an increase in intracranial pressure caused by cerebral oedema, which in addition to reducing cerebral perfusion may cause 'coning' and death, is more common in children.

Assessment of the head-injured patient It is worth stressing again the importance of ensuring that the patient has a clear airway, is adequately ventilated with oxygen, and has a stable circulation.

The conscious level should be assessed formally using the Glasgow coma scale which is shown in Table 3.4. A children's coma scale can be used for children under the age of four, although it has not been validated in the same way as the Glasgow coma scale. The children's coma scale is shown in Table 3.5. It is good practice to itemize the child's response to

Table 3.4 • Glasgow Coma Scale

		Score
Eye opening		
	Spontaneous	4
	To speech	3
	To pain	2
	Nil	1
Best motor response		
	Obeys commands	6
	Localizes stimuli	5
	Withdraws	4
	Abnormal flexion	3
	Extensor responses	2
	Nil	1
Verbal response		
	Orientated	5
	Confused	4
	Inappropriate words	3
	Incomprehensible words	2
	Nil	1
Verbal response modified for small children		
	(appropriate words or social smile)	
	Fixes and follows	5
	Cries but consolable	4
	Persistently irritable	3
	Restless and agitated	2
	None	1

each of the following three assessments: eye opening, motor response, and verbal response.

The pupils should be examined for size and reactivity. A unilateral dilated pupil may indicate raised intracranial pressure requiring immediate neurosurgical action. Local trauma to the eye may also cause a dilated pupil, and a few people have naturally unequal pupils. The eyes themselves should be examined for trauma or haemorrhage which may indicate a base-of-skull fracture.

Look around the eyes for bilateral periorbital haematomas (raccoon eyes) which suggest a base-of-skull fracture or direct facial trauma. Similarly, Battle's sign (bruising over the mastoid process) suggests a base-of-skull fracture. The fundi are usually normal, as papilloedema takes some while to develop in raised intracranial pressure. However, fundal haemorrhages are seen particularly in children who have suffered from the 'shaken child' syndrome.

The nose and ears should be examined for evidence of CSF leak, which also indicates the possibility of a base-of-skull fracture.

The scalp itself should be observed and palpated for haematomas and depressions suggesting a skull fracture.

Finally, the neurological system should be assessed, looking for laterality in tone, movement, and reflexes.

Management of head injury

Deteriorating conscious level If the ABCs are under control, then a deteriorating conscious level suggests increasing intracranial pressure due to either cerebral oedema or an intracranial haematoma. The neurosurgeon must be contacted immediately and a CT scan arranged. The patient should be hyperventilated to a $p\text{CO}_2$ of 28 mmHg, and there may be some benefit in nursing in the 30° head-up position. In patients with signs of developing coning, an infusion of intravenous mannitol should be given at a dose of 0.5–1 g/kg. This should preferably be done only after neurosurgical confrontation.

Convulsions Phenytoin is a useful drug for seizures induced by head injury as it has less sedating effects than diazepam. The dose is 18 mg/kg intravenously over 20 minutes with appropriate monitoring for cardiac irregularities and hypotension which may be caused by this drug.

Indications for neurosurgical consultation

- Deteriorating conscious level
- Focal neurological signs (including focal convulsions)
- Evidence of depressed fracture
- Evidence of penetrating injury
- Evidence of basal skull fracture
- Coma score of less than 12

Indications for urgent airway control and ventilation in the head injured patient

- Unconscious patient with Glasgow coma scale of 8 or less
- Need for airway protection (e.g. facial injuries)
- Inadequate ventilation
- To allow hyperventilation in cases of increasing intracranial pressure

An anaesthetist or experienced senior emergency physician should undertake rapid sequence induction of anaesthesia with thiopentone and suxamethonium or similar drugs. Emergency intubation by the unskilled should be performed only if the child is at extreme risk.

Spinal injuries

The cervical spine will have been protected when the patient first presented during management of the airway. The rigid collar and sandbags should remain in place until the neurological examination, the local examination, and the radiographic examination are shown to be normal. When examining the back of an injured child, he should be log-rolled with the spine in a neutral position.

Examination of the spine and other relevant organs

1. Airway and breathing: breathing may be compromised in the unusual event of thoracic spinal damage causing intercostal paralysis.
2. Circulation: spinal cord injuries cause hypotension and bradycardia due to reduced sympathetic nervous stimulation.
3. Neurological examination: laterality in the limbs in response to painful stimuli, and testing of power, tone, and reflexes should be done; test for anal reflexes and tone; priapism in the male indicates spinal cord injury.

4. Abdominal examination: if there is a spinal cord injury the abdominal walls will be flattened and ileus will develop; it will then be difficult to assess intra-abdominal trauma.

5. Urinary system: a spinally injured patient will develop acute retention and require catheterization.

6. Local examination: the neck and back should be examined for wounds, bruising, swelling, pain, and deformity.

Investigations Cervical radiographs will have been taken as part of the primary survey. In some patients thoracic radiographs will also be necessary. A good view is essential to exclude bony spinal injury. The radiograph must show C7. Look for a prevertebral haematoma which would indicate trauma. The retrotracheal space (C6) should not exceed 14 mm and the retropharyngeal space (C2) should not exceed 6 mm, although this may widen if the child is crying. The atlanto-odontoid gap should not exceed 4 mm; if increased, this indicates rupture of the transverse ligaments of the atlas. Flexion or extension views should not be requested by junior staff. A CT scan of the spine may show abnormality even in the absence of a bony injury.

Management Airway, ventilation, and circulation management are described earlier. If a fracture is identified, the neurosurgeon or orthopaedic surgeon should be contacted urgently. The spine should remain immobilized for transfer.

Limb injuries

Unless there is profuse bleeding or evidence of arterial damage, limb injuries can be left until the potentially life-threatening injuries have been dealt with.

Examination

1. Look at both arms and legs for evidence of bruising, wounds, or deformity.

2. Gently palpate for crepitus or abnormal movement.

3. If the patient is conscious, check voluntary movement at all joints.

4. Feel for the pulse distal to any possible fracture site.

5. Examine the skin overlying the fracture—check for viability by noting its colour and whether it blanches on pressure.

6. If the fracture is compound, examine the wound for soft tissue damage and foreign bodies.

7. Test for function of the part distal to the fracture (there may be associated nerve or tendon damage).

Investigations If a fracture is suspected, the limb should be X-rayed in two planes, including the joint above and the joint below. These X-rays are a low priority, and chest, abdominal, and head injuries must all be dealt with first.

Management If a fracture is suspected clinically, splint the limb. This helps reduce pain, prevent blood loss, and prevent fat embolism.

Check arterial pulses before and after any manoeuvre, i.e. X-ray or reduction. If a distal pulse is absent, call for urgent orthopaedic help. The fracture must be reduced immediately by traction with analgesia.

All compound injuries should be covered. A saline- or beta-dine-soaked gauze is ideal as this helps stop the wound drying out. Alternatively, use clingfilm as this allows the wound to be viewed without contamination. If bleeding is profuse apply a pressure bandage, but monitor the distal circulation and do not allow the patient to leave the department without ensuring that someone in the surgical team knows that a pressure bandage has been applied.

If the injury is compound, give tetanus toxoid if the patient has not received a booster within the last 10 years. Also give intravenous antibiotics, for example flucloxacillin and ampicillin or a cephalosporin. Refer the patient to the orthopaedic department.

Crush injuries

The crush syndrome develops when muscle has been crushed for a length of time, for example if a child is buried under fallen masonry. Muscle breakdown occurs which releases acid myoglobin. When the crush or pressure is released this is carried in the circulation throughout the body. Renal failure is the consequence. Immediately after the pressure is released the child may become shocked and urine output decreases. The limb itself will appear swollen, red, and blistered. Crush syndrome is often fatal. If a crush injury is suspected, an intravenous line should be started and normal saline (20 ml/kg) given to initiate a diuresis. Give intravenous morphine as the limb will be very painful. Monitor ECG for hypercalcaemia. Sepsis is often associated with a more serious prognosis, and so give prophylactic antibiotics (for example flucloxacillin and ampicillin) and be meticulous about wound care.

Amputations

Type of amputation   Clean amputations are the most suitable for reimplantation, but some degloved amputations of fingers and some crush or avulsion amputations can be reimplanted with good functional result. Partial amputations may also benefit from microsurgical procedures.

Care of the amputated part for transfer   The amputated part should be put in a dry polythene bag and placed on top of a bowl of ice with several layers of gauze between the ice and the part. Do not place the part under ice and do not allow direct contact between the part and the ice. Do not put the part and the ice in the same polythene bag. If the amputated part freezes reimplantation is not possible.

Care of the patient   Resuscitate the patient if necessary. Wrap the stump in a sterile dressing and elevate to stop the bleeding. Try to avoid using artery clips to achieve haemostasis as these will damage the vessels. (Use local pressure to stop bleeding with elevation of the limb.) Refer to the nearest plastic surgery centre for reimplantation.

Transfer of injured patients

Once resuscitated, stabilized, and examined, critically injured children will often be transferred to a specialist centre for further treatment. There is often physiological deterioration when patients are transferred from one hospital to another, and so steps must be taken to prevent this.

It is essential to secure the airway, ensure adequate ventilation, and maintain intravascular volume, temperature, and cerebral perfusion pressure during transfer. As much time as necessary should be spent preparing the child as quality of transfer is better than speed.

Transfer check list

1. Adequate sedation or pain relief.
2. Intermittent positive pressure ventilation with full neuro-muscular paralysis.
3. Oximetry and capnography to monitor the ventilation.
4. Adequate secure vascular access.
5. Equipment box with resuscitation drugs and fluids.
6. Heat conservation equipment.
7. Full patient records, charts, and radiographs.
8. Ensure that parents are fully informed.

The patient should be accompanied by an experienced person with skills in airway management and vascular access.

Emergency practical procedures

Needle thoracocentesis
Equipment
- Cleansing swabs.
- Large over-the-needle intravenous cannula (16 gauge or larger).
- 20 ml syringe.

Procedure

1. Identify the second intercostal space in the mid-clavicular line on the side of the pneumothorax.
2. Swab the chest wall with cleansing swab.
3. Attach the syringe to the cannula.
4. Insert the cannula vertically into the chest wall just above the rib below, aspirating all the time. If air is aspirated, remove the needle leaving the plastic cannula in place.

Tape the cannula in place and proceed to chest drain insertion as soon as possible.
If a pneumothorax is not present, there is a risk (10–20 per cent) of causing one. Therefore, any patient who has had this procedure must have a chest radiograph and will require chest drainage if ventilated.

Pericardiocentesis
Equipment
- ECG monitor
- 20 ml syringe

- 6 inch over-the-needle cannula (16 or 18 gauge)
- Skin-cleansing equipment

Procedure
1. Swab the xiphoid area with cleansing material.
2. Attach the syringe to the needle.
3. Puncture the skin 1–2 cm below the left side of the xiphoid junction at a 45° angle.
4. Advance the needle towards the tip of the left scapula aspirating all the time and watching the ECG monitor for signs of myocardial irritation. Once fluid is withdrawn, aspirate as much as possible leaving the cannula in the pericardial sac for further aspiration should tamponade recur.

Intraosseous infusion
Equipment
- Cleansing material
- Intraosseous needle
- 5 ml syringe
- 50 ml syringe
- Infusion fluid

Procedure
Identify the infusion site. In the tibia this is on the anterior surface 2 or 3 cm below the tibial tuberosity. In the femur it is on the anterolateral surface 3 cm above the lateral condyl. Cleanse the skin over the chosen site. Insert the needle at 90° to the skin. Advance the needle with a pushing and twisting motion until a 'give' is felt. This means that the cortex has been penetrated. Attach the 5 ml syringe and attempt to aspirate. This is not always possible. Infuse normal saline. If this passes in easily and there is no swelling of the surrounding tissues, the needle is in the bone marrow. The infusion fluid must be pushed in under pressure. It will not run in under gravity.

Needle cricothyrotomy
- Intravenous cannula and needle or cricothyrotomy cannula over needle
- 10 ml syringe
- Y-connector and oxygen tubing
- Oxygen source

Procedure

Place the patient in the supine position. The cricothyroid membrane is identified by palpating between the thyroid and crycoid cartileges. Cleanse the skin. Stabilize the trachea and insert the needle and cannula through the cricoid membrane at a 45° angle, caudally aspirating all the time. When air is aspirated, advance the cannula over the needle and withdraw the needle. Attach the cannula to an oxygen flowmeter via a Y-connector. The oxygen flow rate in litres should be set at the child's age in years. Ventilate by occluding the open end of the Y-connector with a thumb for one second, but passive exhalation takes longer and at least four seconds should be allowed for this. This procedure is not a definitive airway but will buy time until an ENT surgeon can safely perform the surgical airway.

Continuous assessment

During the secondary survey, while different systems are being assessed, it is important to continue to review the child's condition as a whole in case of further deterioration.
Many severely injured children's lives would be saved by
(1) *getting experienced senior help early*
(2) *avoiding hypoxia—intubate and ventilate early*
(3) *treating hypovolaemia vigorously.*

Further reading

1. American College of Surgeons (1988). *Advanced Trauma Life Support Course core course manual.* American College of Surgeons, Chicago, IL.
2. Advanced Life Support Group (1993). *Advanced paediatric life support—the practical approach.* BMJ, London.
3. Mayer, T. A. (ed.) (1985). *Emergency management of paediatric trauma.* W. B. Saunders, Philadelphia, PA.
4. Coran, A. G. and Harris, B. H. (ed.) (1990). *Paediatric trauma: Proceedings of the 3rd National Conference.* J. B. Lippincott, Philadelphia, PA.
5. Alpar, E. K. and Owen, R. (ed.) (1988). *Paediatric trauma.* Castle House, Tunbridge Wells.

CHAPTER 4

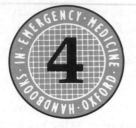

Minor trauma

Wound management

● History   Examination   Management of wounds

One of the most common reasons for a child attending an A & E department is a wound. The treatment given will vary with the type of wound. The main points to be considered are the following.

● Is the wound suitable for primary suture?
● Is there any damage to deep structures?
● Are there foreign bodies in the wound?
● Is the wound dirty?
● Is the wound suitable for management in the A & E department?

If possible the parents should be allowed to accompany the child throughout all procedures.

History

1. Time elapsed since injury—ideally, wounds would be sutured within six hours of having been sustained. After six hours, the skin cells at the edge of the wound may be non-viable. The wound edge will require trimming if

primary suture is to be successful. The exception is a scalp wound in which there is usually an excellent blood supply.

2. Cause and mechanism of the injury, i.e. knife wound, glass, etc. Think about how the wound was caused and what implications this may have. For instance, glass or knife wounds, although insignificant on the surface, often penetrate into deeper tissues causing nerve, vessel, or tendon damage. Wounds inflicted with some force may have caused a deeper injury, such as a broken bone.

3. Possibility of a foreign body—wounds inflicted by glass may contain glass fragments. Other materials, for example thorns, wood splinters, etc., may cause infection later if not removed.

4. Medical history—for example a bleeding disorder. Specific treatment will be required (see Chapter 13).

5. Drug history—for example patients on steroids may have a higher incidence of wound breakdown and infection.

Examination

1. Examine the wound. Decide whether it is clean and suitable for suture, or dirty (see p. 74). Look for areas of skin loss. Gently open the wound for an approximate assessment of its depth. Think what deeper structures may be involved.

2. Palpate the wound for presence of a foreign body.

3. Check movement distal to the wound. Any loss of movement may indicate tendon or nerve damage. This problem usually needs to be referred to the orthopaedic department for further treatment.

4. Assess sensation distal to the wound. A moderately sharp instrument, i.e. an opened-up paperclip, can be used rather than a needle which might frighten the child. If you suspect any loss of nerve function refer the child to a plastic surgeon (even very distal wounds may warrant repair).

5. Feel for the distal pulse and assess circulation. A laceration of an artery may need repair and therefore should be referred to a vascular, general, or plastic surgeon. Digital arteries and nerves run closely adjacent to each other, and

so if there is digital arterial bleeding also suspect nerve damage.

6. Radiographs should be taken of all wounds caused by glass, but a full wound assessment must also be made. All glass is relatively radio-opaque, but whether or not glass fragments show on the radiograph depends on various factors, i.e. the size and orientation of the foreign body, the X-ray exposure, and the radiodensity of the tissues. Glass may easily be obscured by overlying bones. In order to show a glass foreign body it is often necessary to ask for soft tissue and/or tangential views. If a glass foreign body is present, it should be removed unless it is extremely small and difficult to access.

Management of wounds

Abrasions   These are wounds which have removed the surface of the skin but have not penetrated into the deep tissues. They should be very thoroughly cleansed as any residual dirt will leave tattoo marks. Lignocaine gel (2 per cent) applied 15 minutes before cleaning, will produce some analgesia. Smaller abrasions may have lignocaine infiltrated beneath them before cleaning. Beware of toxicity from lignocaine; calculate maximum dose first (Table 4.1). Extensive or facial abrasions will

Table 4.1 • Maximum safe dose lignocaine 1% at different ages (maximum safe dose of lignocaine is 3 mg/kg, 1% lignocaine contains 10 mg/ml)

Age of child	Maximum safe dose 1% lignocaine (ml)
6 months	2
12 months	3
2 years	3.5
3 years	4
4 years	4.5
5 years	5
6 years	6
7 years	7
8 years	7.5
9 years	8
10 years	9
11 years	10
12 years	11

usually need to be cleaned under general anaesthesia. Use forceps and a small brush to remove embedded dirt. When the wound is completely clean apply a dressing (except on the face). Very clean wounds should have a non-adherent dressing such as paraffin gauze applied. Wounds which were very dirty or those caused in a dirty area (for example in the garden) may have an antiseptic added to them, i.e. spray with povidone–iodine or cover with a paraffin gauze impregnated with chlorhexidine or povidone–iodine. The parents should be advised to leave the dressing on for about a week (earlier removal would be painful and may remove new tissue) and to keep the dressing clean and dry. Patients with minor abrasions can usually be discharged to the care of the GP.

Lacerations Do not attempt any repair unless you are entirely confident to do so. The following wounds are not suitable for suture in the A & E department.

1. Extensive wounds—may need general anaesthetic.
2. Deep wounds with tendon, nerve, or arterial damage—refer to the appropriate surgical team.
3. Facial wounds—consider referral to the plastic surgeon. Wounds involving foreheads and chins can usually be sutured in the A & E department. Refer large wounds and wounds involving the red margins of the lips and around the eyelids as these need meticulous repair to prevent scarring.
4. Large areas of skin loss or devitalized tissue—refer to the plastic surgeon.

Sutures Suturing small children's wounds is difficult as the child cannot understand what is happening to him. A brief demonstration on 'teddy' may dispel fear.

Wounds which can easily be sutured in the A & E department are those which involve skin only. Decide whether adhesive strips or tissue adhesive may be more appropriate than sutures.

When you have finished suturing it is important to give the parents instructions about the care of the wound, i.e. keep it clean and dry, and check for signs of infection (redness, pain, swelling, and discharge). A printed instruction card may be helpful. Tell the parents when the sutures should be removed and refer the child to the GP or district nurse for this to be done (see p. 76). Lacerations which have been difficult to suture, have had areas of skin loss, or are potentially infected should be reviewed in the A & E department. Advise the parents about signs of infection and tell them to return if concerned.

Adhesive strips These are a suitable alternative to suturing for small superficial wounds. They are not suitable for wounds over a moving part (for example a joint) or where they might easily become damp. The wound must be fresh and clean. The advantages of adhesive strips are that they are painless to apply, do not require any expertise for removal, and do not leave suture marks. However, it is essential that the basic principles of wound management are adhered to and the wound is cleaned and explored adequately. Gaps must be left between the strips to allow for any discharge to escape. Opposition of skin edges should be accurate, and wounds not suitable for suture are unlikely to be suitable for adhesive strips. Tincture of benzoin applied with cottonwool to the skin adjacent to the wound will help the strips to adhere. It may be helpful to use forceps to lift up the skin edges to ensure that they do not roll under and therefore cause the wound to heal poorly. The parents should be instructed to keep the strips clean and dry. They are removed after a similar period of time as sutures, or can be left longer if necessary.

Tissue adhesive This is a modified 'superglue' which will hold together skin edges, provided that there is no tension or movement. The wounds must be superficial. The wound is cleaned and dried and a thin layer of adhesive applied over the wound. The skin edges are held together for one minute while the glue sets. The reaction produces heat which may be uncomfortable for the patient, but otherwise the procedure is pain free. The wound can be left exposed and the glue, which is biodegradable, will hold for several days. The method is ideal for small scalp wounds and some facial lacerations.

Antibiotic prophylaxis Although all the wounds which are seen in the A & E department are contaminated with bacterial organisms, prophylactic antibiotics are rarely required. If the wound is only superficially dirty, adequate cleansing should suffice to prevent infection. The wound must be repaired so that no necrotic tissue is left to encourage infection, and the wound should not be under tension as this may compromise the vascular supply and hence healing. If the wound is clean and has a good blood supply, there is only a small risk of infection and this can be treated later if it occurs. However, prophylactic antibiotics should be considered in the following cases.

1. Wounds which have been very heavily contaminated with dirty material, for example mud from a field or garden.

2. Penetrating wounds where it is impracticable to clean the whole wound tract without extending the wound and causing more tissue damage (for example wounds caused by rusty nails).

3. Bites (see p. 78).

4. Wounds in which there has been a delay in presentation (of more than six hours) where bacterial multiplication may already have occurred.

5. Wounds in which there may be some dead space or areas of poor vascular supply.

Note: Prophylactic antibiotics are no substitute for meticulous wound cleaning and adequate debridement and repair of the wound.

Suitable antibiotics need to be chosen according to the most likely pathogen. Send a wound swab for bacteriological studies so that, on review, the pathogen can be identified and the appropriate antibiotic given.

1. Flucloxacillin is active against staphylococci which are found on normal skin and are a frequent cause of wound infection. It may also be used in conjunction with ampicillin or co-amoxiclav which is a broad-spectrum antibiotic.

2. Co-amoxiclav is ampicillin combined with clavulanic acid and is active against many bacteria, including some anaerobes and the penicillinase-producing organisms. It is particularly suitable for animal bites.

3. Penicillin is used where streptococci may be the suspected organism; it will also kill *Clostridium tetani* (but tetanus prophylaxis is vital).

4. Erythromycin is a useful broad-spectrum antibiotic suitable for patients who are sensitive to the penicillins.

The dose given should be appropriate for the child's age and is usually given orally for five days.

Tetanus toxoid Every child who attends the A & E department with a wound should have their tetanus immunization status checked. Even if the wound is not thought to be tetanus prone it is essential to maintain immunity in case infection occurs in future wounds.

Most children have their routine immunizations, including tetanus toxoid, at two, three, and four months of age (primary course (TTC)) and a booster (TTB) at five years of age. These will provide immunity from tetanus until the child is 15 years old. However, some children may not have received adequate immunizations, in which case Table 4.2 should be used for reference.

Contraindications to tetanus vaccine are as follows:

- acute febrile illness—except in the presence of a tetanus prone wound
- severe reaction to a previous dose.

The community health physician should be informed of children who have received tetanus immunization in hospital so that unnecessary further doses are not given in the community. Also consider whether to give Diptheria and Polio immunization at the same time; if the child has not received the full tetanus course, neither will he be adequately covered against Diptheria and Polio.

Table 4.2 • Tetanus chart

State of immunity	Wound tetanus prone	Requirements
TTC or TTB within 10 years	Yes	Nil*
	No	Nil
TTC or TTB more than 10 years ago	Yes	TTB and human tetanus immunoglobulin
	No	TTB
Incomplete TTC or unimmunized or unknown	Yes	TTC and human tetanus immunoglobulin
	No	TTC

* TTB may be given if the risk is high, for example stable manure.

A tetanus-prone wound has one or more of the following characteristics:

- dirty (i.e. contact with soil or manure)
- puncture wound
- devitalized tissue
- more than six hours old
- clinical evidence of sepsis.

Stabbings If the history indicates a stab wound, be very careful. The innocuous-looking skin defect may conceal serious underlying damage to vital structures. Always take a detailed history with a description of the sharp instrument involved, if possible. If the object is still *in situ*, do not remove it as this may cause torrential bleeding. If the wound track lies near any major vessels, it should be removed in theatre with full resuscitation facilities immediately available. Probing wounds does not always give an adequate indication of the depth of the wound and can be dangerous.

Stab wounds to the chest, head, neck, and abdomen must be treated seriously. Even if the patient appears well, always insert an intravenous line and cross-match blood in case of sudden catastrophic bleeding. These wounds should always be referred for surgical investigation and exploration.

Stab wounds to the limbs should be thoroughly examined and checked for damage to deep structures. Patients may need to be referred to the orthopaedic department for exploration under general anaesthesia. Small shallow wounds with no underlying major structures may be explored and sutured in the A & E department.

Palatal penetration Children may fall while sucking a sharp object such as a pencil. In this case the object may penetrate the hard palate and cause serious damage. There is also a risk of injury to the carotid artery. All penetrating wounds to the roof of the mouth should be referred to the appropriate surgical team for exploration under general anaesthesia.

Puncture wounds

Puncture wounds to the feet are not uncommon. Unshod children may step on a sharp object, or the shoe may be penetrated by a nail. Ask and record what object caused the injury.

Radiographs must be taken of injuries caused by glass, needles, etc. to exclude the possibility of a retained foreign body. If the causative object is unknown it is also wise to take a radiograph. Foreign bodies should be removed, usually under general anaesthesia. Occasionally, the wound becomes infected and this may lead to osteomyelitis or septic arthritis (sometimes due to a *Pseudomonas* infection). Prophylactic antibiotics are not necessary in every case of penetrating wound, but the parents should be carefully warned about the signs of infection and asked to return if they are worried.

Bites

Dog bites Dog bites vary in severity from the trivial to the life-threatening. The actual circumstances surrounding the injury are usually very frightening for both the child and the parents. The dog may cause damage with his teeth or claws. These wounds are always contaminated with bacterial organisms and often become infected. Because of the risk of infection, dog bites should not be sutured on the day of injury. The wound should be thoroughly cleaned and explored using local or general anaesthesia as necessary. The wound is left unsutured, an antiseptic dressing (for example paraffin gauze impregnated with chlorhexidine or povidone–iodine) applied, and the patient given prophylactic antibiotics. After three or four days the wound is reviewed and assessed for infection. If the wound is clean, it can be repaired if necessary by delayed primary suture or closed with steristrips. Before suturing or steristripping the wound, a millimetre or less of skin should be excised from each skin edge. The fresh skin edges can then be opposed and sutured as a fresh wound. It is essential that no tension is placed on the wound which may prevent it healing. Undermining the skin edges may help accurate apposition. The antibiotics are continued and the wound reviewed at regular intervals of about two or three days.

Facial wounds may leave ugly scars if left for delayed primary suture. As the face has a good blood supply, most dog bites of the face can be sutured early under antibiotic cover. These cases should be referred to the plastic surgeon unless they are very minor.

Cat bites Cat bites usually cause less tissue damage than dog bites, but create puncture wounds which are frequently infected with anaerobes such as *Pasteurella multocida*. Co-amoxiclav should be given for prophylaxis and review in two days is necessary.

Human bites The human mouth is very heavily colonized with bacteria, including anaerobes. Human bites should be treated in a similar fashion to dog bites, but they become infected even more frequently. Prophylactic antibiotics against anaerobic bacteria should be given (for example co-amoxiclav). The child may have been bitten by someone who is a hepatitis B carrier or who carries the HIV virus. Hepatitis immunoglobulin and vaccine should be given. At present there are no recommendations for HIV prophylaxis. The wound should be thoroughly cleansed to reduce the amount of contamination.

Non-accidental injury should be considered (p. 155).

Insect bites These may cause a local allergic reaction with redness, swelling, and itch. If there is no evidence of infection, 1 per cent hydrocortisone cream applied topically will provide relief. Sometimes the child appears with a rash. Pointers that this might be due to a crop of insect bites are the linear nature of the line of red spots and the distribution, usually on the lower legs or around the lines made by elastic in clothing. Extensive numbers of bites may cause intense itching and an oral antihistamine can be given. Some bites become infected, and there may be an ascending lymphangitis or cellulitis around the bite. If this occurs, penicillin V or erythromycin should be given. A local abscess may need to be treated by incision and drainage.

Insect stings Wasp stings are usually a very minor problem, although they may occasionally cause an anaphylactic reaction. Symptomatic treatment is usually sufficient. If the child is stung in the mouth there may be some swelling but this usually subsides rapidly. However, a sting in the throat may cause enough swelling to obstruct the airway, and the child should be observed in the A & E department for two to three hours after being stung. If the sting is on the hand, this should be elevated in a sling for 24 hours.

Bee stings are more likely to cause an anaphylactic reaction. If it is a simple sting remove the embedded sting with a needle or forceps. Treat symptomatically, but the same caution with oral stings applies as above (for anaphylaxis see p. 40).

Soft tissue injuries

Soft tissue injuries are bruises, pulled muscles, etc. They are often trivial, but some of the more serious injuries need to be treated with as much respect as a fracture (and may be difficult to differentiate from such). A sprain is an example of this type of injury (see p. 110).

Bruises A bruise is a bleed into the underlying skin or soft tissues. It can be classified as an ecchymosis, which is a bleed into the skin, or a haematoma, which is a more extensive bleed into the soft tissues.

1. Ecchymosis—this presents as a red–purple area on the skin. As the bruise ages it turns yellow–green with the altered blood pigment. It is important to determine the cause of the bruise, always bearing in mind the possibility of non-accidental injury. If assault is likely, document the size and appearance of the bruise carefully in the notes in case a police statement is required. An ecchymosis needs no treatment other than reassurance. Spontaneous bruising may be a sign of leukaemia, bleeding disorder, septicaemia, or non-accidental injury.

2. Haematoma—this usually presents as a swelling with an overlying bruise, and with pain on touching the affected part. Again, it is important to take an adequate history to determine the cause. Check the distal circulation and sensation. The child will probably be more comfortable if the area is supported by firm bandaging and elevated. Very large haematomas may be aspirated. This must be done as soon as possible after the injury as clotted blood is difficult to remove. Use a large gauge needle (i.e. 16 g) and a strict aseptic technique. Choose the most dependent part of the haematoma to allow for drainage. Blood or occasionally yellow serious fluid can be aspirated. Apply a firm bandage after aspiration to prevent re-accumulation of blood. The child should usually be reviewed in the A & E department. If the haematoma is unusually large or increases markedly in size, consider the possibility of a bleeding disorder such as haemophilia.

Fingertip injuries

• History   Assessment   Management

Fingertip injuries are a common sight in any A & E department and causes distress to the parents and the child.
Although the initial damage often looks alarming, most fingertip injuries heal very well, resulting in a normal finger. Amputated fingertips regrow spontaneously with remarkably good
results.

History

The most common aetiology is for the child's finger to be
trapped in a door or door hinge. It is important to determine
the exact cause of the injury so as to assess the risk of infection. Injuries which happen in the garden or are caused by
bites are particularly prone to infection.

Assessment

The child will be in pain and an early priority is to give analgesia. First look at the finger and examine the finger distal to
the injury. Test for sensation and function of the tip. Once this
has been documented, a digital nerve block can be inserted
before proceeding further. This will provide analgesia whilst
further examination and treatment are carried out.

Examination   Check for the following.

1. The site of the avulsion or injury—this will determine the
   management of the injury and the prognosis.

2. The degree of bony involvement—look to see if any bone is
   exposed or if there is any bone deformity. Occasionally
   there is an open dislocation of the finger when the articular
   surfaces of the bone are seen.

3. Nail damage—the nail may be completely or partially
   avulsed.

4. Sensation and function of the tip give an indication of the
   viability of the distal part.

Management

X-ray the finger—to check for bone damage and the length of bone remaining.

Crush injuries proximal to the distal phalanx—these should be referred to the orthopaedic department for further treatment.

Re-implantation—this should be considered for any finger injury proximal to the distal interphalangeal joint, although a more distal injury in a thumb may be considered suitable.

Injuries distal to the distal interphalangeal joint—these can usually be managed in the A & E department. Check that the initial ring block is still providing complete analgesia before proceeding. Some more complicated injuries and injuries in small children may need to be repaired under general anaesthesia. Cleanse the area thoroughly. Check the nail for damage. If the nail is almost completely avulsed then remove it. Occasionally the base of the nail is pulled away from the nail bed. This should be replaced by repositioning it under the nail fold. This helps prevent deformity of the new nail. The finger must be meticulously cleaned and any dead tissue debrided. If the tip is partially avulsed, any deformity should be corrected and the tip positioned in its correct state. This should be fixed in place by one or two absorbable sutures. It is not advisable to use many sutures for a fingertip as they tend to tear the skin. Adhesive strips are an excellent alternative. If the tip is completely avulsed, the distal end can be left without skin cover as the skin will eventually grow over and provide new cover. After the surgical repair is complete a paraffin gauze dressing should be applied and covered with a dry finger dressing. The dressing should not be removed until the child is reviewed after one week. (Removing the dressing, which often sticks, may cause damage by pulling off partially healing areas and is also very painful. There is usually no need to see the wound earlier.) The appearances at one week are often still poor, but the parents should be reassured about the eventual outcome. The child should be reviewed at weekly intervals until the tip is healed. If the bone is damaged or exposed, prophylactic antibiotics should be given, for example ampicillin and/or flucloxacillin, or erythromycin if the child is penicillin sensitive.

Subungual haematoma—blood under the nail causes quite severe pain which can be relieved if the pressure is released. Using a flame-heated paperclip, puncture the nail in the centre over the haematoma. Blood will then drain through the hole. This is only effective if done within 24 hours of the injury, as old blood will have clotted.

Soft tissue infections

• **Abscess   Cellulitis   Lymphangitis   Paronychia Ingrowing toe-nail**

Abscess

An abscess is a pus-filled cavity; the usual contaminating organism is a staphylococcus. The organism enters through a breach in the skin which may have been caused by minor trauma or an insect bite. An abscess may present at any site. Perianal and axillary abscesses seen in adults are rare in children but may be seen in adolescents.

History

1. Possible cause of the abscess—this might indicate the type of infection, i.e. an insect bite may be infected with streptococci.

2. How long has it been present? This may indicate the severity of the infection.

3. How painful is it and can the child sleep at night? Tense pus is extremely painful.

4. Any previous history of abscesses? The child might need investigation for an underlying immune deficiency.

5. Ask about symptoms of thirst and polyuria—occasionally an abscess is a presenting sign of diabetes.

6. Previous medical history—diabetics and children on steroids are likely to have abscesses which are slower to heal.

7. Any treatment already given for this abscess, for example antibiotics—these will alter the symptoms and signs, and might produce a walled-off abscess which does not heal but which is less invasive.

Examination

1. Size of the abscess—only small abscesses are suitable for incision and drainage in the A & E department. Large abscesses are too painful and need curetting adequately.

2. Is it fluctuant? If the abscess is pointing or is fluctuant, it is ready for incision and drainage.

3. Site of the abscess—be wary of infected lumps in the neck as these may be infected branchial or thyroglossal cysts which need surgical referral.

4. Take the child's temperature and examine for lymphadenopathy—these indicate whether the child is toxic, i.e. has a systemic spread of the abscess infection which will require systemic antibiotic treatment.

5. Urine test—for sugar to exclude diabetes.

Management

1. Fluctuant abscesses should be incised and drained using general anaesthesia.

2. Large abscesses need surgical referral.

3. Antibiotics should not be given unless the child is toxic or there is any cellulitis around the infected site. Antibiotics do not adequately penetrate pus and the end result is a partially treated abscess which is not fluctuant and is resistant to treatment.

4. A pus swab should be obtained in case further antibiotic treatment is necessary post-operatively.

5. The patient should be reviewed in 24–48 hours to check that the abscess is settling.

Cellulitis

Cellulitis is an infection of the subcutaneous tissues. The organism is usually a streptococcus or staphylococcus. The child usually presents with a painful red swollen area, usually on a limb. There is often a small cut or graze. The infected area will be inflamed, swollen, and tender. The regional lymph nodes may be enlarged. The child's temperature should be taken. If the child is toxic and unwell, he should be admitted to hospital for parenteral antibiotics. If the infection is less severe, he can be managed at home. The affected part should be rested and elevated. A high arm sling is useful for an arm. If a leg is affected it should be elevated on a foot stool. An antipyretic–analgesic, for example paracetamol, should be given. Antibiotics should be prescribed, usually ampicillin plus flucloxacillin or penicillin V. Erythromycin can be used for penicillin-sensitive patients. Blood cultures should be taken to identify the pathogen. The child should be reviewed daily to check that the infection is subsiding. If vomiting occurs, the oral antibiotics will not be effective, and admission and parenteral antibiotics may be needed.

Lymphangitis

Lymphangitis is an infection extending along the lymphatic channels to the local lymph glands and is almost always streptococcal in origin (occasionally staphylococcal). The patient will usually have a break in the skin (caused by minor trauma) which is the portal of entry for the infection. Ascending from this is a red line. The local glands will be palpable and the patient pyrexial. Oral penicillin plus an antipyretic, for example paracetamol, is usually sufficient for treatment. The limb should be elevated and rested. The patient should be reviewed 24 hours later. The lymphangitis should resolve within 24–48 hours.

Paronychia

Bacteria can enter through the base of the nail folds and cause inflammation of the surrounding tissues. A painful red

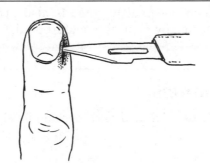

Fig. 4.1 • Incision of paronychia.

swelling forms on one side of the base of the nail and develops into a pus-filled blister. It is easily treated by incision either through the area which is pointing or by a vertical incision just lateral to the base of the nail (Fig. 4.1). A digital nerve block should be used. The finger should be cleaned and dressed. Antibiotics are only required if there is marked cellulitis.

These infections must be distinguished from a herpetic whitlow, in which there are more discreet small papules or blisters and a longer history. Herpetic whitlows require no treatment but are very painful and often recurrent.

Ingrowing toe-nail

Ingrowing toe-nails are common in adolescent boys. The aim of treatment is to relieve the infection and prevent recurrence. The patient presents with a painful red swelling adjacent to the medial distal edge of the toe-nail. Mild cases can be treated by elevating the edge of the nail involved and putting an iodine-soaked wick underneath it. (This procedure is painful and may require digital nerve block.) This allows the pus to drain and enables the nail to grow long and away from the skin edge. More severe cases may need all or part of the nail removed. This allows free drainage and healing of the skin before the nail regrows. If the ingrowing toe-nail is recurrent, excision of the lateral part of the nail and phenolization of the nail bed produces good results. Nail avulsion can be done with a good digital nerve block, or it may need a general anaesthetic. To prevent recurrence the patient should be advised to wear broad-toed shoes and to cut the nail straight across. Good personal hygiene is also necessary. Most cases are best treated by referral to a chiropodist.

Foreign bodies

• Ears   Nose   Inhaled and ingested foreign bodies

Ears

The parents might notice the child putting the object into the ear and come immediately to the A & E department. Sometimes, however, the incident is not seen, and some days later the parents notice the object or the child admits to the incident. Examine the ear carefully using an auriscope. If the object is easily visible and the child is cooperative, it may be possible to extract the material. It is preferable to use a hook to draw the object out (but be careful when going posteriorly to avoid damaging the drum). Forceps may push the object further down the canal. If the attempted removal is unsuccessful then the child should be referred to the next ENT clinic.

Nose

Foreign bodies in the nose are a more urgent problem as they may be inhaled and therefore should usually be removed the same day. Ask the child (if old enough) to blow his nose, occluding the unaffected nostril. This may dislodge the object. If it is possible to hook the object out, then do so. A large syringe may be useful to suck out food debris. If these procedures are unsuccessful, the child should be referred without delay to the ENT surgeon.

Inhaled and ingested foreign bodies

See p. 148 and p. 185.

Nasal problems

• **Trauma Epistaxis**

Trauma

The nose is usually damaged by a fall onto the face or by a direct blow. The child may have an epistaxis. The bridge of the nose is usually swollen and tender. Important points to note in the examination are as follows.

1. The presence or absence of a septal haematoma—in this case the nose is blocked and a cherry-red swelling is apparent inside it. This is an ENT emergency, as, if left untreated, the nasal septum may become necrotic and the nose will collapse. The treatment is drainage of the haematoma under general anaesthesia.

2. Nasal deformity—if the nose is bent, it will need straightening. This is usually done about one week after the injury when soft tissue swelling has subsided and it is easier to correct the alignment of the nose. This is done under general anaesthesia by the ENT or plastic surgeon.
3. Septal deformity—occasionally the septum is deviated to one side. Again, this should be referred to the ENT surgeon within a few days.

Most nasal injuries do not require an X-ray (except when there is a skin break on the nose and one needs to determine whether there is a compound fracture present). In children under five years old the nasal bones are mainly cartilaginous and do not show up on an X-ray; after this age the importance of the injury is based on clinical rather than X-ray findings.

Epistaxis

Children quite frequently have small nosebleeds. The aetiology may be trauma, allergy, infection, or foreign body. The bleeding is usually venous, and unless the child has a bleeding disorder simple measures such as pressure should cause it to stop. Ask the child to hold the soft part of the nose between his fingers for at least 15 minutes. He should breathe through the mouth and sit with the head forward.

Occasionally the bleeding is more persistent and further treatment will be necessary. A nasal pack can be inserted by someone experienced in the procedure. An anterior nasal pack has the disadvantage that there may be a persistent posterior nasal bleed. This can be seen by looking down the child's throat. The child should not be discharged whilst there is persistent bleeding. Assess the child for blood loss by checking the pulse and blood pressure, and looking for pallor and sweating (remember that more than 25 per cent of the blood volume must be lost before there are clinical signs of shock). The child may need to be admitted for observation and occasionally may need transfusion.

Dental problems

● **Mouth and tongue injuries**

Traumatic avulsion of a tooth is a common problem. It should be replaced as soon as possible. If this is done, the tooth will usually reattach and remain viable. If the tooth is brought with the patient to the A & E department, place it in normal saline. The dentist on call for the hospital should be informed immediately. Best results are obtained the earlier the tooth is re-implanted, and this should be within four to six hours. Outside hospital it is recommended that the tooth is cleaned using tap water. It should then be placed in a container of milk. Older children may be able to keep the tooth in the mouth adjacent to the gum. Even milk teeth merit re-implanting as their presence ensures correct development of the underlying second tooth.

The child may also present with the teeth pushed forwards or backward after a fall. These should be repositioned. This can often be done in the A & E department by standing behind the child and applying pressure. If this is unsuccessful, the child should be referred to the dental surgeon immediately. If the tooth is loose, this can usually be treated by the child's own dentist. It is safe to wait overnight, unless the tooth is very loose and there is a danger of its coming away completely and being aspirated. It may be possible to glue the loose tooth to adjacent teeth with tissue adhesive until definitive dental treatment can be arranged.

Toothache is less common in children than in adults. It may be due to a carious tooth which will be obvious on inspection. The child should be given some paracetamol and referred to his own dentist. The pain may be due to a dental abscess, in which case there may be swelling and tenderness around the tooth and swelling of the face. This should be treated with oral penicillin V and analgesia, for example paracetamol elixir. If something stronger is needed, try Ibuprofen syrup. The child should then visit his own dentist the following day. Occasionally one can see the abscess pointing into the mouth. The child should be referred to the on-call dental surgeon for treatment.

Mouth and tongue injuries

Lacerations to the mouth and tongue occur after falls or direct blows to the face. Examine the mouth, tongue, and teeth carefully. Despite moderate bleeding, the damage may only be slight. Most lacerations involving the oral mucosa can be left without suturing. The parents should be warned that a yellow slough may appear around the laceration. This is a local colonization from the common flora in the mouth and does not need treatment. The child should be encouraged to eat normally. Cold foods, i.e. ice-lollies and ice-cream, will help numb the pain and reduce swelling. If the laceration extends over the vermilion border this should be very carefully sutured as any slight irregularity will leave an ugly scar. Consider referring the child to the plastic surgeon. If there is a small laceration extending through from the oral mucosa to the skin, the skin wound should be sutured as normal leaving the mucosal wound open. Large wounds should be referred to the plastic surgeon for suturing of the muscle layer. Lacerations to the tongue only need suturing if they extend over more than one-third of its surface or if there is continued bleeding. The tongue is very difficult to suture, and referral to a dental or plastic surgeon may be necessary.

Injuries to the palate may occur, particularly if the child falls whilst running with a sharp object in the mouth (see p. 77).

Needlestick injuries

Children may find abandoned needles and suffer a puncture injury. The injury is usually trivial, but parents are usually concerned about the risk of HIV and hepatitis B infections.

The current recommendation is that children who suffer a needlestick injury receive an accelerated course of hepatitis B vaccine.

No prophylaxis is recommended for HIV infection, but serology can be undertaken three to six months post-injury—an initial blood sample should be taken for comparison, after counselling.

It is important to stress to parents that the risk of being

infected with either virus from a needlestick injury is extremely small. Both viruses, and particularly HIV, are sensitive to extremes of heat and humidity and do not survive to infect in these circumstances.

Eye problems

● **Infections   Foreign bodies in the eye   Conjunctival abrasions   Eye injuries**

Infections

Eye infections are common and may present at any age.

1. Stye—this is a localized infection of the eyelash follicle, usually staphylococcal in origin. There is a small discrete swelling with erythema on the border of one eyelid. If possible, remove the offending eyelash to help the infection drain. Chloramphenicol eye ointment 1 per cent (or gentamicin 0.3%) should be applied twice a day until the infection resolves. Systemic antibiotics are rarely necessary.

2. Blepharitis—a more generalized swelling of both eyelids may occur. This is often allergic in origin, associated with hay fever or asthma, or allergies to shampoo or soap. The symptoms are relived by removing the allergen, for example using non-perfumed products, and using an antihistamine if the symptoms are severe. An infective blepharitis also occurs with crusting of the eyelashes. This should be treated with chloramphenicol eye ointment 1 per cent (or gentamicin eye ointment 0.3%).

3. Conjunctivitis (see p. 236).

4. Orbital cellulitis (see p. 236).

Foreign bodies in the eye

The child will say that he feels something in his eye. This may be very painful and there will be a reluctance to open the eye for examination. It is important to make sure that the child can keep still so that the eye can be examined under a bright light. The eyelid should be everted to check for the presence of a foreign body stuck under the tarsal plate. If there is a history of a high velocity radio-opaque foreign body entering the eye, for example hammering metal, an X-ray should be taken. If the child is cooperative, use amethocaine eye drops for analgesia and attempt to remove the foreign body with a damp cotton wool bud (do not attempt this unless you are confident in your ability to do so). Small children will need a general anaesthetic. After removal give the child chloramphenicol eye drops or ointment (or gentamicin 0.3%) for a few days to prevent infection.

Conjunctival abrasions

Again, the child might feel as if there is something in the eye or have pain in the eye. Stain the eye using fluorescein eye drops. Any epithelial damage will stain and show up as a fluorescent green area. Superficial abrasions can be treated by giving chloramphenicol eye drops (or gentamicin 0.3%) and covering the eye with a pad. The lesion should be reviewed and restained after two days, by which time it will probably have healed. Occasionally a herpetic dendritic ulcer will be seen on staining. This has a branching appearance. The child should be referred to the ophthalmologist.

Eye injuries

Most eye injuries are potentially serious, particularly if there has been any possibility of a penetrating injury, and should be referred to the ophthalmologist. An eye patch should be put over the eye to prevent eye movement and analgesics given if necessary.

Head injuries

- **History   Examination   Investigations   Management**

Injuries in the apparently well and conscious child are described in this section (see also p. 59). Head injuries account for about 10 per cent of child attendances with trauma at an A & E department. Many of these injuries are trivial, but it is important to detect the case which may have a complication.

History

1. Degree of trauma—a useful guide to the potential seriousness of the injury is to assess the forces involved in the accident. Children who have been involved in road traffic accidents, fallen downstairs, or fallen from a height are much more likely to have sustained significant brain injury; they may also have other injuries apart from those to the head.

2. Child's condition immediately after the accident. Was there a period of unconsciousness? Did the child have a fit? Did he cry immediately? A few seconds loss of consciousness does not affect the child's prognosis. However, loss of consciousness of over a minute suggests a more serious head injury.

3. Vomiting—many children vomit once after almost any degree of head injury. Persistent vomiting is more significant.

4. Drowsiness or irritability—ask whether the child has fallen asleep at an unexpected time or whether he has cried excessively or been fretful.

5. Visual symptoms—young children would not complain of double vision but might give some indication that their vision is blurred or different from usual. This is evidence of concussion with an inability of the brain to function normally.

6. Headache—a small child may only indicate the presence of pain by excessive crying. An older child might complain of a pain in the head.

7. Length of time since the injury—children are sometimes brought days after an injury with a history of being unwell and vomiting. This may be due to a totally unrelated illness (for example otitis media), the symptoms of which the parents relate to the head injury. It is unusual to have a delay of more than a few hours before the symptoms of a head injury occur; hence symptoms occurring several hours or days after the injury may be related to something else. Children fall more frequently when they are ill, and it may be difficult to decide whether the head injury is causing the symptoms.

Examination

1. Assess the child's level of alertness. Bear in mind the time of day, since the child would be likely to be sleepy late at night, or a baby might often be asleep during the day. See how easily the child can be roused if sleepy.

2. Check the cervical spine for any tenderness or restricted movement.

3. Examine the scalp for evidence of injury. Look for lacerations or haematomas. Palpate the area around the injury for tenderness or evidence of bone deformity which might indicate a depressed fracture (this may be masked by haematoma).

4. Check the nose and ears for any evidence of bleeding or fluid leak. If fluid is present it may be CSF and would indicate a fracture of the base of the skull. Also look behind the ears for bruising (Battle's sign) which would also indicate a fracture of the base of the skull.

5. Orientation—an older child can be asked standard questions about time, person, and place.

6. Neurological examination—a full range of tests is not always necessary. Observe the child's limb movements, tone and power, and coordination. Test the limb reflexes. In a small child the parents may be the best guide of the child's behaviour.

7. Pupil reflexes and fundal examination—shine the torch in the child's eye to check for pupil size and reaction. Fundal examination should be performed. Look for papilloedema. This is unlikely to be present in the short term, even with raised intracranial pressure. Also examine for retinal haemorrhages which might suggest child abuse (see p. 157).

8. Take the child's temperature and look in the ears and down the throat. Evidence of an underlying upper respiratory tract infection might help explain symptoms which are out of keeping with the degree of trauma. If the child has a temperature or headache give him some paracetamol before sending him for X-ray. The child often looks better when seen later. Continue neurological observation whilst awaiting X-ray results.

Investigations

Skull X-ray The following guidelines are suggested by the Royal College of Surgeons:

- loss of consciousness or amnesia at any time
- neurological symptoms or signs
- CSF or blood from nose or ear
- suspected penetrating injury or foreign body
- scalp bruising or swelling
- difficulty in assessing the patient, i.e. very young child
- alcoholic intoxication

A minor scalp laceration is not an indication for X-ray, but X-rays should be used for a deeper laceration showing periosteum.

In addition, consider X-ray in the following:

- following substantial trauma, road traffic accident, fall from a height, heavy blow (for example a golf club)
- Other findings suggesting basilar skull fracture (haemotypanum, Battlo's sign, supra orbital haomatoma)
- depressed area on palpation (ask for tangential views)
- non-mobile infants, as the likelihood of non-accidental injury is higher and accidental injury lower in these infants
- children in whom an adequate history is not available.

Brain injury and skull fracture are two separate and sometimes coexistent entities. There may be severe brain injury in an unconscious child with no skull fracture, and conversely most skull fractures will not cause any problems. The presence of a skull fracture is an indicator of possible complications following a head injury. However, children are more likely than adults to suffer complications without a skull fracture as their skulls are softer and may deform, causing brain damage without a fracture. Babies may become shocked from bleeding into a scalp haematoma (sometimes without a fracture).

Cervical spine X-ray Always consider this with a significant head injury.

CT scan This should be considered in any child with neurological symptoms or signs, or decreasing conscious level (see p. 61).

Management

Criteria for admission following 'minor' head injury

1. Skull fracture
2. History of loss of consciousness of a minute or more.
3. Drowsiness.
4. Persistent vomiting (many children vomit once or twice after a head injury and then stop; this is not an indication for admission).
5. Neurological symptoms or signs, for example severe headache, convulsions.
6. Lack of supervision at home.
7. Clinical evidence of basilar skull fracture.
8. Substantial trauma, for example fall from a first-floor window.

If the child is alert, has no skull fracture, and can be observed overnight by sensible adults, he can be discharged. Sometimes a further short period of observation in the A & E department may be sufficient to make the final decision easier.

If the child is discharged, the parents should be clearly informed about the symptoms and signs to look out for, and when to bring the child back to the A & E department for reassessment. It is useful to reinforce the information with written instructions. The parents should be told to wake the child once or twice in the night to make sure that he is rousable. They should return if the child begins vomiting, if he complains of a headache unrelieved by paracetamol, visual disturbance, or if he becomes unexpectedly drowsy, unusually irritable, ataxic, or has a convulsion.

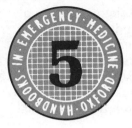

CHAPTER 5

Fractures and orthopaedic problems

Key points in fractures and orthopaedic problems

1 Children's injuries differ from those of adults. They are less likely to sprain a ligament and more likely to sustain a greenstick or avulsion fracture. Radiographs should be taken more readily than in adults.

2 Injuries which involve the growth plate must be treated carefully as later growth disturbance may occur. However, a greater degree of fracture angulation can be tolerated in children compared with adults as growth will remodel the bone.

3 A limp should be thoroughly assessed as there are several possible underlying causes which may lead to problems if untreated.

Fractures

- **Types of fracture specific to children   Management of fractures**

Children have different types of fractures from adults as

97

growing bones differ from the mature skeleton. Children's bones are less brittle than those of adults and often deform to produce buckle or greenstick fractures. Comminuted fractures are unusual. A child's ligaments are relatively stronger but laxer than those of adults, and so sprains are unusual and growth plate fractures are more common. Injuries which involve the growth plate must be treated carefully as they may lead to growth disturbances.

Types of fractures specific to children

Greenstick or buckle fracture This is an incomplete fracture of the bone. The cortex is disrupted on one side and intact on the other. Symptoms and signs are often minor. The fracture may only show as a small irregularity of the cortex on the radiograph. They heal very well, but immobilization in plaster of Paris is usually required for pain relief. Some greenstick fractures can be appreciably deformed and may need reduction.

Growth plate fractures The growth plate is a cartilaginous disc between the epiphysis and metaphysis. Fractures in this area are described according to the Salter–Harris classification (Fig. 5.1).

Type I—epiphysis separates completely from the metaphysis.

Type II—the line of fracture travels through much of the plate before passing through the metaphysis and detaching a triangular metaphyseal fragment. This is the most common injury.

Type III—the fracture line passes along the growth plate for a variable distance before entering the joint through a fracture of the epiphysis. This is very rare.

Type IV—the fracture line passes from the joint surface across the epiphysis and growth plate, and into the metaphysis.

Type V—These are crush injuries of the growth plate. There is often very little to see on the X-ray at first, but deformity appears months or years later because bone growth has stopped. This type is rare.

Special attention should be paid to types III and IV because of their intra-articular component. Other fracture categories are as described in adults.

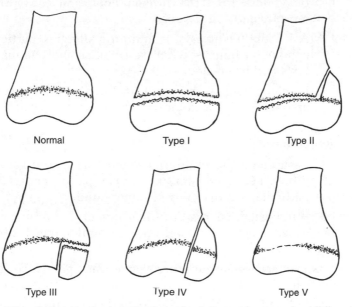

Normal Type I Type II

Type III Type IV Type V

Fig. 5.1 • Salter–Harris classification of epiphyseal fractures in childhood.

Management of fractures

History

1. Assess the degree and nature of the trauma. The history may suggest the likelihood of a fracture, for example a fall from a height or a road traffic accident is likely to produce serious injuries, some of which may not initially be obvious. Knowledge of the actual mechanism of injury, for example whether a rotatory force was applied, may be helpful when reducing the fracture.

2. Pain—the amount of pain that the child feels will vary from slight (for example in greenstick fractures) to severe (in many displaced fractures).

3. Function of the affected part—note whether the child can walk on the affected leg or use the damaged arm. Most fractures will lead to a significant loss of function.

4. If a fracture is compound, ask about any bleeding apparent at the scene of the accident. There may be considerable

blood loss from the broken bone and the surrounding muscles and soft tissues.

5. Ask about tetanus status and drug allergies, particularly in compound injuries where antibiotics and tetanus prophylaxis will be needed.

6. Previous trauma—frequent fractures might suggest consideration of non-accidental injury or osteogenesis imperfecta.

Examination

1. Resuscitate the child if needed. Check the general condition, i.e. blood pressure, pulse, pallor, conscious level, particularly if the injury is compound.

2. If indicated, i.e. road traffic accident, fall from a height, or possible non-accidental injury, examine the child for other injuries.

3. Tenderness—examine the area very gently so as not to cause further pain. Palpate around the affected part.

4. Deformity—this may be immediately apparent, but children can have a significant fracture with minimal outward signs.

5. Swelling—the soft tissues surrounding a fracture are usually also damaged. This, together with the deformity and bleeding from the fracture itself, will cause swelling. With certain fractures, such as a greenstick fracture, there may be little or no swelling.

6. Crepitus and abnormal movement—these may be present at the site of a fracture. However, eliciting these signs is painful and should not be done intentionally.

7. Loss of function—ask the child to move the affected part in all directions. Do not do this if the fracture is obvious.

8. Examine for neurovascular damage distal to the injury. In particular, check and record the distal pulse. Absence of pulse indicates that there has been arterial damage and immediate treatment is required. Check and record sensation.

9. Assess soft tissue damage—sometimes the soft tissue element of the bony injury is as significant as the fracture itself. Check for ligamentous damage using a stress test. If

a fracture is compound, assess the amount of skin damage and look for muscular tears.

10. Examine the limb and joint above and below the injury site as there may be damage to these areas as well.

X-rays The decision as to whether or not to X-ray the injured part can be difficult. There is a need to balance the fact that fractures can occur with minimal clinical signs against the risks and costs of unnecessary radiation. If the history of the degree of trauma is sufficient to cause a fracture in a symptomatic patient (i.e. road traffic accident, falls downstairs, etc.), X-rays should be taken. If the child shows any one of the clinical signs of a fracture (i.e. tenderness, swelling, loss of function, deformity, crepitus, or abnormal movement), a radiograph should be taken. Radiographs should usually be taken in two planes and should include the joint below and the joint above the injury.

Treatment The aims of treatment are to relieve pain and to restore the functional anatomy of the part. Initial splinting will prevent further deformity, provide some relief from pain, and help minimize further blood loss.

1. Resuscitate—some fractures, especially those of the femur and compound fractures, may bleed significantly and the child will need an intravenous infusion. Associated severe or potentially serious injuries for example chest or abdominal injuries should be treated first (see Chapter 3).

2. If there is no distal pulse palpable, immediate action is required. If the limb is deformed, reduction of the fracture may restore the blood flow. This can be done in an emergency in the A & E department using Entonox for analgesia. Restoration of circulation is a priority before X-ray. Call for urgent orthopaedic help. Always check the arterial pulses before and after splinting.

3. Immobilize the affected part—for example a broad arm sling for the forearm or a padded splint for a leg.

4. Analgesia—if necessary this should be given prior to X-ray. In the case of finger injuries, digital nerve block may suffice. An opiate (for example morphine or pethidine) is required for displaced or compound fractures. Paracetamol is usually sufficient for children with greenstick fractures.

5. Reduction—if the fracture is displaced it will need reduction. In most departments this procedure is carried out by orthopaedic staff. Sometimes a minor degree of deformity is acceptable in a younger child who has a greater potential for bone remodelling. The reduction can be closed, usually by simple traction, or open when operative methods are used. Prolonged traction is sometimes needed, for example for fractures of the femoral shaft. Most reductions in children require a general anaesthetic.

6. Maintenance of reduction—the fracture must be held in position until it heals. In some cases, for example a single fracture of a middle metatarsal, there is adequate support from nearby structures without external fixation. Usually plaster of Paris is used. The fracture should be held by plastering the joint above and the joint below the fracture to prevent movement at the fracture site. If the limb is swollen, a circumferential plaster should not be applied as further swelling may lead to distal ischaemia. In this case the child should be admitted overnight for elevation of the limb and delayed plastering. A half-plaster (black slab) is used for temporary support until the swelling diminishes. Whenever a plaster has been applied, the patient should be reviewed the following day for a plaster check.

7. If the injury is compound, check tetanus status and give intravenous antibiotics, for example ampicillin plus flucloxacillin or a cephalosporin. Cover the open wound with a sterile dressing. These injuries should be referred to the orthopaedic department immediately.

8. Follow-up—most patients will be referred to the fracture clinic for follow-up. Local guidelines should be followed.

Elbow effusions

The child presents with a history of a fall on to the elbow or outstretched hand. The elbow may be swollen. There will be generalized or local tenderness. Movements will be restricted. X-rays show a positive fat pad sign, but no fracture can initially be detected. The fat pad is a radiolucent area seen on the radiograph anterior to the humerus at the elbow. If there is an effusion (of either blood or fluid) in the elbow, the fat line is pushed forward. The lucent line stands out from the humerus. This is known as the positive fat pad sign. About a third of cases will eventually turn out to have a fracture not detectable on the original X-rays. Other causes are a haemarthrosis or traumatic effusion. Rarely, the trauma is a precipitating or exacerbating factor for another cause of joint swelling, for example septic arthritis. Any child with an elbow effusion should be treated with a collar and cuff and reviewed in an A & E department or fracture clinic to assess the elbow further and to check for recovery of movement.

Pulled elbow

This usually occurs in children under five years of age (usually one to three years). The presenting symptom in this condition is that the child will not use his arm. He may complain of pain in the shoulder, elbow, or wrist. The parents may be worried that the arm is dislocated or broken.

The diagnosis is suggested by the history. There has usually been a pull or fall involving the arm. Often the child has nearly fallen and an adult has held the arm to help pull the child up. The child then stops using his arm and holds it to his side. The mechanism of the injury is that the radial head (which is poorly formed at this age) has slipped through the annular ligament at the elbow. A pulled elbow is very easily reduced by flexing the elbow to 90° and then supinating the forearm while extending the elbow. Usually a 'click' can be felt or head, and the child starts using his arm normally. An X-ray of the arm is not necessary unless there is any doubt that the child may have actually fallen or sustained direct trauma to the arm. A pulled elbow will look normal on a radiograph. The child may not always start using the arm immediately, particularly if there has been some delay before reduction. Allow the child to play in the A & E department before reassessing. Most children will have recovered within half an hour. If the child is still not using the arm, then put it in a collar and cuff sling and review the child the following day. Warn parents that a pulled elbow may recur (in either arm) but that the child will grow out of the problem. There will be no long-term sequelae. Ask them to avoid pulling on the child's arms.

Table 5.1 ● Management of specific fractures

Region	History	Examination	X-ray	Treatment	Special complications
Clavicle	Fall onto outstretched hand Direct blow onto shoulder	Tender along clavicle Palpable deformity Arm movement painful	Fracture often middle third May be angulated Easily seen later when callus forms	Sling or collar and cuff under clothes Mobilize when pain free	Lump at site of fracture may persist for some months
Humerus	Fall onto outstretched hand or elbow Direct blow	Tender at site Bruising Movement of shoulder and elbow	May fracture through neck of humerus with fracture separation Fractured shaft may be siral or transverse (NB normal epiphysis may look like a fracture)	Collar and cuff (uses arm as traction Occasionally U-slab plaster	Radial nerve damage Check active extension of fingers
Elbow: supracondylar fracture	Fall onto hand with elbow bent	Elbow swollen and tender Pain on movement	May be undisplaced Often distal humeral fragment displaced backwards and twisted inwards Positive fat pad sign	Displaced fractures need reduction Undisplaced fractures held in collar and cuff	Volkmann's ischaemic contracture Check radial pulse before and after X-ray and manipulation Early orthopaedic review
Elbow: fracture of lateral condylar epiphysis	Fall onto hand Elbow may dislocate and spontaneously reduce	Elbow swollen Lateral tenderness Movement painful Active wrist dorsiflexion limited	Lateral humeral fragment may be grossly displaced Incomplete fracture more difficult to see	Accurate reduction of displaced fracture under general anaesthetic (? open reduction needed) Undisplaced, collar and cuff	

Injury	Cause	Signs	X-ray	Management	Complications/Notes
Elbow: separation of the medial condylar epiphysis	Fall onto hand Occurs before epiphysis fused (under 16 years) Association with lateral dislocation of elbow	May be obvious deformity and swelling Medial tenderness	Medial epicondylar epiphysis may be twisted or shifted downwards Fragment may still be in joint	If displaced needs reduction (may be open) If undisplaced, collar and cuff	Ulna nerve damage Check sensation in lateral fingers
Fracture of head and neck of radius	Fall onto outstretched hand (may be in valgus position	Deformity and swelling may be slight or absent Pain on rotation of elbow and tenderness on lateral side	Transverse line distal to growth plate Proximal fragment may be tilted Radial head may show vertical split, a lateral fragment displaced distally, or comminuted fracture Positive fat pad sign	If large displaced fragment or if head of radius tilted more than 15° refer for manipulation Undisplaced fractures can rest in collar and cuff	
Proximal radius and ulna	Fall or direct blow to the forearm	Often obvious fracture with deformity swelling and tenderness	Breaks may be transverse or oblique and at same or different levels There may be angulation	May need reduction depending on degree of angulation Undisplaced fractures need an above-elbow plaster May need hospital admission for swelling	Single fractures of the radius/ulna are unusual Look for possible dislocation at radio-ulnar joints, e.g. Monteggia fracture (fracture of upper third of ulna and dislocation of head of radius (or Galeazzi fracture (fracture of lower third of radius and dislocation of interior radio-ulna joint)

Table 5.1 ● Continued

Region	History	Examination	X-ray	Treatment	Special complications
Distal radius and ulna:	Fall onto outstretched hand Delay in presentation not unusual as signs often minimal	Swelling of wrist Tenderness to palpation Decreased wrist movement	Slight angulation of cortex of one or both bones May show in one plane only	Plaster of Paris backslab applied for short period of time for pain relief and protection	Will heal well
Distal radius	Fall onto dorsiflexed hand	Wrist often swollen with obvious deformity	May be fracture separation of lower radial epiphysis (tilted backwards and/or medially May also fracture or crush radial metpahysis	Accurate reduction if displaced Short arm plaster of Paris	Crushing of metaphysis may lead to abnormal growth of arm
Carpal scaphoid	Fall onto outstretched hands Common in adolescents uncommon in children under 12 yrs	Wrist may look normal Palpate carefully for tenderness in anatomical snuff box Pain on hyperextension of wrist	Take in several planes as fracture difficult to see (scaphoid views) Usually across waist (proximal pole or tubercle may also be damaged) X-rays at 10–14 days may show fracture more clearly owing to bone resorption	Plaster of Paris in scaphoid position If clinically suspected ffracture X-ray again in 10–14 days	Avascular necrosis of distal part (which receives its blood supply from the proximal part and this is disrupted by a fracture) Risk of arthritis
First metacarpal	Fall or hyperextension injury	Swelling or tenderness around joint	1. Transverse fracture distal to carpo-metacarpal joint, distal	Reduction under general anaesthetic Held in Bennett's	

	Mechanism	Clinical features	X-ray	Treatment	Complications
		Thumb may be shortened	portion may be displaced and/or impacted 2. Fracture dislocation with oblique fracture extending into joint—Unstable	plaster	
Other metacarpals	Direct blow to hand, or twisting or punching injury	Hand often bruised and swollen. May be visible lump. Assess movement of fingers for any rotational deformity	Fracture of one or more metacarpals spiral or transverse. Fracture necks usually transverse but the head may be angulated	Undisplaced or slightly displaced fractures need no treatment and active movement should be encouraged. Displaced fractures may need reduction. Fractures of several metacarpals may need plaster of Paris	Loss of knuckle (with fractures of head metacarpal). Extensor lag when moving fingers
Phalanges	Many types of mechanism. Direct blow. Angularity force. Stubbing of the finger. Often associated with sports injuries	Swelling and tenderness. Look for angulation or rotation of finger (best assessed by asking child to make a fist). Check lateral stability of each joint for ligamentous injury	Will show site of fracture, degree of angulation and joint involvement. Small chip fractures adjacent to a joint may indicate a significantly injury	If no angulation or rotation, strap adjacent fingers together (neighbour strap); this provides lateral support but allows joint movement. Review at 7–10 days. Refer spiral or angulated fractures	Swelling may persist for some weeks. Encourage movement to prevent stiffness
Phalangeal dislocations	Direct trauma	Often obvious. Check neurovascular status in distal fingers	This will show dislocation and any associated fracture	Reduce dislocation as soon as possible (digital nerve-block) then neighbour strap fingers	After reduction check for ligamentous stability of joint

Table 5.1 • Continued

Region	History	Examination	X-ray	Treatment	Special complications
Femur	Severe force needed, e.g. road traffic accidents (although infants may fracture more easily)	Usually mid-thigh swelling with some deformity Unable to bear weight Check peripheral pulses	Will show the fracture site, type, and degree of deformity (NB May also have pelvic fracture)	Place in traction splint (e.g. Thomas's splint) before X-ray The child will need to be admitted	IV fluids/blood may be required owing to blood loss in the thigh May damage femoral artery (check pulses)
Patella	Significant fall Direct blow Crushing injury to the knee	Knee swollen and held flexed Movement painful Ask child to raise leg to check extensor muscle function	The patella may fracture without displacement or be comminuted (NB Bipartite patella is a normal finding	Refer for admission Dislocated patellas need reduction and post-reduction splinting	
Proximal tibial spine and tubercle	Hyperextension injury to the knee Avulsion of tubercle due to insertion of tubercle extensor muscles)	Knee is held flexed and is swollen Cannot be extended	Lateral view will show avulsed tibial spine Fracture of tibial epiphysis is often displaced forward Patella will be high	Some fractures may need reduction and aspiration of the associated haematoma	
Tibia and fibula	Fall Direct trauma Twisting force to leg whilst foot stationary	May be obvious deformity Palpate for bony tenderness Check neurovascular status	Include ankle and knee joint Spiral or transverse fracture Single or both bones affected Assess angulation	May need reduction Refer for admission and elevation Above-knee plaster of Paris	Compartment syndrome Post-traumatic swelling compromises the vascular supply to the foot

Ankle	Inversion injury Direct blows Fall from height	Unable to bear weight Swelling Bony tenderness Neurovascular status Test ankle joint stability	X-ray in two planes Check integrity of ankle mortise (widening on one side) may indicate unstable fracture)	If undisplaced, below- knee plaster of Paris Refer if displaced
Os calcis	Fall from height or jump	Unable to bear weight Heel swollen and tender Ankle movement	Need os calcis views Fractures are chip, crush, split (NB Sever's disease, osteochondritis of os- calcis)	Because of swelling most cases are admitted for elevation prior to plaster of Paris May have associated lumbar spine fracture

Sprains

  • **Sprained ankle**   **Knee injuries**

A sprain is a stretch or tear of a ligament, commonly occurring around the ankle, although this term may be used to describe finger, wrist, or shoulder injuries. Sprains are less common in children than in adults because the young child's ligaments are extremely strong and the trauma instead causes damage to the bony attachment of the ligament around the epiphyseal plate. Therefore it is more important that an X-ray of the associated bone is taken when a sprain is suspected in children.

Sprained ankle

The usual mechanism is an inversion injury to the ankle (the child usually says that he went over on his ankle) which may or may not have caused a fall. A stress is put on the lateral talo-fibular ligament and occasionally on the anterior ligament. This results in the stretching or tearing of the ligament, and there may also be damage to the bony attachments to the fifth metatarsal or lateral malleolus.

History   Ask about the exact details of the injury. This will help in assessing which ligaments may be involved and the type of injury that may be seen. Is the child able to bear weight? This will help indicate the severity of the injury. Ask about the child's interest in sport. A sprained ankle in a child who takes part in competitive sport may have significant implications for his training and achievements.

Examination

1. Swelling—the degree of swelling is not an indication of the severity of the sprain. It will depend on many factors, such as the length of time since the injury (most swelling occurs after 24–48 hours), the amount of walking done, and whether the ankle has been held dependent.

2. Bony tenderness—feel for the ligamentous insertions and the bones around the ankle. Bony tenderness is a definite indication for X-ray.

3. Stability—the amount of 'give' compared with the unin-

jured ankle can be assessed by putting a lateral stress on the ankle joint. However, this may be too painful to be performed adequately. A useful test is the anterior draw test: the ankle is held with one hand, and the foot is held and pulled forward. This causes little pain and it is easier to compare the amount of forward 'give' with the normal ankle.

Management   X-rays should be taken of most ankle injuries in children as there may be an associated fracture. If the child cannot bear weight an X-ray of the ankle must be taken (if there is a fracture see Table 5.1). Occasionally a small fragment of bone is seen on X-ray just distal to the lateral malleolus. This is an avulsion fracture and should be treated as a severe sprain rather than a more serious fracture. If the ankle appears unstable, orthopaedic referral is needed. The possibilities for treatment are operative repair (rarely needed), immobilization in a plaster case, or active mobilization. If the ankle is stable, the aim is to encourage the child back to full mobility as soon as possible. A firm support bandage, i.e. a tubular elastic bandage, is helpful initially as the child will feel more able to walk on the leg. If the ankle is very swollen, the leg should be elevated above hip height for periods during the day, for example 1 hour three times a day. A cold compress helps to relieve the swelling. Encourage the child to walk on the ankle as soon as possible. Sporting activities should be delayed until the child has no limp, and then restarted gradually.

Knee injuries

Serious knee injuries are more often a problem for the adolescent than the smaller child. Sometimes an underlying abnormality, i.e. Osgood-Schlatter's disease or chondromalacia patellae, is precipitated or becomes apparent following an injury.

History   It is important to gain an accurate description of the mechanism of injury as this indicates the most likely component of the knee to be damaged, i.e. a twisting injury on a fixed lower leg would indicate a meniscal injury.

1. Time elapsed since injury—the knee will often become swollen. If this occurs rapidly, it indicates bleeding into

the knee. A slower rate of swelling is more suggestive of post-traumatic oedema.

2. Previous knee symptoms—might indicate an underlying knee problem.

3. Sporting history.

4. Previous medical history—haemophiliacs may present with a swollen knee due to haemarthrosis.

Examination

1. Look at the knee for evidence of swelling and deformity, and note the position in which the knee is held.

2. Palpate the knee. Feel for areas of tenderness which would indicate regions of damage, for example the joint line or ligamentous insertions.

3. Check for swelling. Is there an intra-articular effusion? Test this by feeling for an area of fluctuation around the patella or a patellar tap. There may be extra-articular swelling.

4. Put the knee through its usual range of movements both actively and passively. It should be able to be fully extended and should flex until the heel of the foot touches the thigh.

5. Test for any degree of adduction or abduction with the knee straight. Compare with the other knee. There is usually only a minimal degree of give. Any more than this indicates ligamentous laxity. Repeat with the knee flexed to 30°, again testing the medial and lateral ligaments.

6. Flex the knee to approximately 90° and pull the tibia forward from the femur to check for anterioposterior glide. This would indicate damage to the anterior cruciates (again, compare with the other knee).

7. Rotate the lower leg with knee flexed to different positions. If this is painful it may indicate meniscal damage. Ask the child to raise the leg with the knee in full extension. This assesses the quadriceps expansion and patellar tendon function.

Management Unless the injury is thought to be trivial an X-ray should be requested. Fractures are often difficult to detect clinically and other conditions, for example Osgood–Schlatter's disease, may also be diagnosed. Indications for immediate orthopaedic referral are as follows:

- avulsion of tibial tubercle
- moderate to large effusion
- any degree of instability of the knee
- bony abnormality
- inability to bear weight
- inability to extend the knee fully

These may indicate serious intra-articular pathology which are best assessed soon after the injury.

If none of the above signs are present, the knee should be supported in an elasticated tubular bandage (usually used double). Crutches can be used if the child has difficulty bearing weight. The child should be reviewed in the A & E department or fracture clinic, after about five to seven days.

The limping child

- **Important points in the history   Examination
  Investigations   Referral   Osteochondritis**

A common problem in the A & E department is a child who has developed a limp or gait abnormality. In many of these cases no cause is found and normal gait recovers spontaneously. However, there are several conditions which need to be considered:

- soft tissue or bony trauma
- irritable hip
- osteomyelitis
- septic arthritis
- Perthes' disease
- slipped femoral epiphysis
- neuromuscular disorder, for example Guillain–Barré disease (p. 224) or cerebellar ataxia.

The history and examination should be directed at confirming or excluding the above conditions.

Important points in the history

1. The age of child—some conditions are more likely to occur

in certain age groups, for example slipped femoral epiphysis usually occurs in adolescents. Irritable hip is more common in children under five years of age.

2. History of recent trauma—this will suggest soft tissue or bony damage as a cause of the limp. However, underlying conditions are sometimes unmasked by trauma or, since children often fall, the parents may recall a minor injury which they think is the cause of the problem.

3. History of recent illness (for example sore throat or viral infection). An irritable hip is thought to follow a viral infection two to three weeks previously. A superficial infection may suggest secondary osteomyelitis or septic arthritis. Rubella often causes a mild transient arthritis which may present as a limp.

4. How long has the child been limping? A history of several day's duration might indicate a condition with slow onset, for example Perthes' disease, whereas septic arthritis is more acute.

5. Previous medical/surgical problems—a history of osteogenesis imperfecta would obviously lead to an examination for fractures. In a haemophiliac child one might expect to find a haemarthrosis.

Examination

Examine both legs completely. A limp may be caused by problems with any area from the foot to the hips. Observe the child lying down and the position in which the leg is held. Look for areas of swelling and redness. Palpate the whole leg for tenderness. Examine the knee, testing for an effusion. If an effusion is present, is the knee warm or cool? Put the knee through active and passive flexion and extension. Examine the hip for areas of warmth or redness. Carefully assess flexion, extension, internal and external rotation, and abduction and adduction of the leg. Note if the movements are painful or limited. Watch the gait if the child is able to walk. In addition note the following.

1. Child's temperature—if the child is systematically ill, this would suggest an infectious cause for the limp, such as osteomyelitis or septic arthritis. (A normal temperature does not exclude these conditions.)

2. Child's general condition—look for evidence of other affected joints which may indicate an arthropathy.

3. Look for evidence of other injuries or bruising—bear in mind the possibility of non-accidental injury.

4. Examine the child neurologically—depressed lower limb reflexes will suggest Guillain–Barré syndrome.

Investigations

Take X-rays of both hips and any other area of the limb in which bony damage is clinically suspected. The hip X-ray in irritable hip may show widening of the joint space, although this is better demonstrated on an ultrasound scan. Ultrasound may be preferred as it will show an effusion in the hip joint which would confirm the presence of hip pathology and indicate orthopaedic referral. Look carefully at the femoral epiphysis for the ragged appearance of Perthes' disease and the appearance of a slipped femoral epiphysis. Also, take blood for the following:

- a white cell count and erythrocyte sedimentation rate (ESR) (or equivalent)
- blood cultures if the child is pyrexial.

Note These may all be normal in early osteomyelitis or septic arthritis.

Referral

Most children should be referred to the orthopaedic department for further assessment and possible admission. The child may only be allowed home if no abnormality has been found on examination, he is apyrexial and has a normal blood count, and the radiographs appear normal. However, he must be reviewed in 24 hours.

Irritable hip This occurs mainly in children under five years of age. There may be a history of a viral illness two to three weeks prior to development of the limp. The child is usually quite well, but has a definite limp. There is usually some limitation of hip rotation, but there may be very little else to find on examination. X-rays may show an effusion and blood tests should be normal. An ultrasound scan will show the effusion well. Treatment is to rest the limb and sometimes traction. The child may need admission.

Perthes' disease This is a form of osteochondritis of the femoral head which usually occurs in children aged five to ten years. The onset may be gradual. There is no systemic upset. On examination there will often be limitation of movement, especially abduction and internal rotation. X-rays (include a 'frog' position) may show distinctive features, such as flattening, fragmentation, or increased density of the femoral head. Compare both femoral heads on X-ray. The child should be referred to the orthopaedic department.

Slipped upper femoral epiphysis This condition occurs in older children, usually from 10 to 15 years old. The child may be overweight. There may be a history of trauma. On examination there is usually reduction in abduction and internal rotation. X-rays should be taken with a lateral or 'frog' view of the hip. (The Anterioposterior view may be normal). This will show the epiphyseal slip. Surgical intervention may be needed and the child should be referred to the orthopaedic surgeon.

Osteomyelitis and infective arthritis Infection can occur in any age group and is potentially very serious. The child may be toxic and pyrexial with a raised white cell count and ESR (but these may also be normal). Examination will show the leg to be held externally rotated and abducted and the child will be reluctant to move it. Radiographs are initially normal. The child should always be admitted. In the early stages there may be few clinical signs. Later, local pain and tenderness develop.

Osteochondritis

The osteochondritides are a group of conditions in which there is abnormality of a growing area of bone. They present with pain around the region with some loss of function. The areas commonly involved are as follows:

• metatarsals	—Freiberg disease
• navicular	—Köhler's disease
• lunate	—Kienbock disease
• capitulum	—Panner's disease
• tibial tuberosity	—Osgood–Schlatter's disease
• calcaneum	—Sever's disease

(Osgood–Schlatter's disease may also be due to a traction apophysitis.)

In these areas rapid growth is thought to occur with some resulting deficiency in the blood supply to the bone. Radiographs of the area may show deformity, fragmentation, or increased bone density. In most cases symptoms resolve with rest, but referral should be made for an out-patient orthopaedic opinion.

Osteochondritis dessicans is a particular form of osteochondritis when a fragment of bone actually separates from the main bone. This occurs particularly around the distal femur. In this case the bone may need to be fixed surgically and the patient should be referred.

Arthritis

• **History   Examination   Investigations   Treatment**

A child may present with one or more swollen joints. Commonly fingers, knees, or ankles are involved.

Common causes are trauma and infection; less frequently juvenile arthritis is found.

History

1. Age of child—most of these conditions can present at any age.

2. History of trauma—this would suggest an injury as the cause of the swelling. However, as children often fall, the swelling may be incorrectly ascribed to the injury. Therefore a history of trauma does not exclude other diagnoses.

3. Time since onset—swelling following trauma usually occurs fairly rapidly. Swelling due to sepsis comes on more slowly, but still has an acute time span. In cases of arthropathy the swelling may have been present for several days or weeks.

4. Single or multiple joint involvement—arthritis is the likely diagnosis when more than one joint is involved. The pattern and type of joints affected also help diagnose the type of arthritis present.

5. Previous joint problems—again this might indicate an arthropathy.

6. Recent illnesses, for example exanthema, viral infection, or sepsis. Rubella is frequently followed by an arthralgia in older children. This may also occur after rubella vaccination. Meningococcal infection may also be associated with an arthropathy.

7. Rash—this may be associated with some rheumatological conditions. A child with Henoch–Schonlein purpura usually has arthritis (p. 233).

8. Easy bruising or excessive bleeding—consider a bleeding disorder.

9. Diarrhoea—occasionally a reactive arthritis follows an episode of diarrhoea.

10. Eye symptoms—iritis and uveitis are associated with arthritis. The eye will be painful with some photophobia.

Examination

1. Examine the joint involved. In particular look for a joint effusion or generalized tissue swelling. Feel the warmth and look for redness. Put the joint through a full range of movements to assess function.

2. Examine other joints for similar signs.

3. Assess the child's general condition. Take the temperature and feel the pulse rate. A child with osteomyelitis or septic arthritis may be pyrexial and toxic (although occasionally there are no systemic features). Children with rheumatoid arthritis may also be systemically ill.

4. Look for rashes.

Investigations

1. The joint involved may need an X-ray. Look for fractures. Sometimes a joint effusion may be apparent. In osteomyelitis there may be no initial X-ray changes, but later there is patchy rarefaction of the metaphysis and a periostitis which shows as a thin line parallel to the shaft. Later still, as healing occurs, there is sclerosis and new periosteal bone.

2. White cell count, ESR (or equivalent), and rheumatoid factors may be taken.

3. Other investigations as indicated, for example blood cultures.

Treatment

Trauma   The most common cause of swelling is trauma. If infection and arthritis have been excluded, the affected part needs to be rested and splinted. The patient should be reviewed in 48 hours, and then active mobilization should be encouraged.

Osteomyelitis or septic arthritis   Usually the child is ill with a raised temperature, a rapid pulse, leucocytosis, and a raised ESR. Occasionally, particularly in the early stages, the child may look misleadingly well. If infective causes are suspected, the child must be admitted. The child holds the part very still. It will look more red and swollen as the disease progresses. Tenderness is felt over the bony metaphysis. In septic arthritis the child will not move the joint because of spasm. The child should be referred to the paediatric or orthopaedic department immediately for further investigation and treatment. Delay in treatment may lead to chronic osteomyelitis, altered bone length, suppurative arthritis, or metastatic infection.

Arthritis   Juvenile arthritis can present in several forms and as it is unusual may be overlooked for some time. Early recognition is important as treatment may prevent later disability. The presentation may be with single or multiple joint involvement, or a series of joints over a period of time. The systemic form occurs in younger children. There is a rash and generalized toxic symptoms; joint involvement is not always initially apparent. Transient arthritis can also occur after a viral illness, in particular rubella. This may also occur two to three weeks after rubella immunization. Arthritis with a purpuric rash on the lower limbs is Henoch–Schonlein purpura (p. 233). The child with suspected arthritis should be referred to the paediatrician for investigation and treatment.

Sickle cell crises   See p. 238.

Further Reading

1. MacRae, R. (1989). *Practical fracture treatment* (2nd edn). Churchill Livingstone, Edinburgh.
2. Grech, P. (1981). *Casualty Radiology*. Chapman and Hall, London.
3. Keats, T. E. (1988). *Atlas of normal roentgenographic variants that may simulate disease* (4th edn). Year Book Medical Publishers, Chicago, IL.

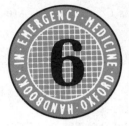

CHAPTER 6

Burns and scalds

Key points in burns and scalds

1 Thermal injuries may be extremely painful and analgesia should be a priority after resuscitation.

2 Children with injuries of over 10 per cent of their body surface always require admission and intravenous fluids.

3 Inhalation injury is potentially fatal and its possibility should be actively considered.

4 Even trivial burns should be followed up as they may develop complications.

5 Consider the possibility of non-accidental injury.

Epidemiology

• First aid treatment

Burns and scalds are the most common cause of accidental death in children in England and Wales after road traffic accidents. Most deaths are the result of house fires, and many victims are under five years of age since they are incapable of

121

making their own escape. The main causes of house fires are as follows:

- matches found and used by children
- cigarettes discarded by adults
- faulty room heaters.

The immediate cause of death in house fires is usually suffocation due to the reduction in ambient oxygen, carbon monoxide poisoning, and toxic smoke emitted from burning household furnishings.

Scalds and contact burns are common in children under five years old; burns from playing with matches, fires, or flammable liquids are more common in older children, particularly boys.

First aid treatment

The emergency management of a minor burn or scald should be to run cold water over the affected part for five to ten minutes, cover the wound with a clean non-fluffy dressing, such as a tea-towel, pillowcase, or clingfilm, and bring the child to the A & E department. No creams or ointments should be used.

Initial assessment of the patient

- **Cardiopulmonary status Pain relief History Area of injury Thickness of burn Sites of burn Intravenous infusion Other injuries**

Cardiopulmonary status

Assess cardiopulmonary status, particularly the airway and breathing. If the patient is shocked or in respiratory failure, as shown by weak, rapid pulse, low blood pressure, poor capillary return, depressed conscious level, respiratory difficulty, or cyanosis, cardiopulmonary resuscitation as described in Chapter 2 should be instituted. Few patients, even with major burns, will be shocked on arrival, but they can deteriorate quickly. At least hourly observations of pulse, respiration rate, blood pressure, and urine output should be made. Early intubation may be needed in victims of fires, inhalation of steam, or scalds or burns of the face and mouth (see inhalation injury (p. 128).

Pain relief

Burns and scalds are extremely painful and pain relief is a priority. Patients with major burns will need intravenous morphine (0.1 mg/kg) provided that there is no contraindication such as a history of head injury. This dose can be repeated if the child is still in pain. The injection should be given slowly, preferably into an infusion. Intramuscular morphine is poorly absorbed in the severely injured child but can be used after small burns if there is severe pain and distress. Patients with minor burns should be given oral analgesics, such as paracetamol 10 mg/kg, and cold compresses should be applied to the wound whilst the burn is being assessed.

History

A detailed history of the thermal injury and the patient's past medical history should be sought. Full details of the accident, including the time at which it occurred, are important in assessing the severity of the injury and fluid requirements. Information can be gained from relatives, ambulance personnel and firemen.

The current tetanus immunization status should be noted. If the circumstances of the history are inconsistent with the extent or degree of the burn, the possibility of child abuse should be considered (see Chapter 8).

Area of injury

The size of the burn should be assessed using Table 6.1 and Fig. 6.1. It is important that this is done accurately, as it will determine the amount of intravenous fluid given and whether or not the child is admitted to hospital. Table 6.1 gives the relative dimensions, at different ages, of the areas of skin shown in Fig. 6.1. It will be noticed that the relative proportion of head size diminishes as the child grows, while that of the leg assumes a higher percentage. One side of a child's palm and closed fingers cover approximately 1 per cent of his body surface area.

Burns covering more than 10 per cent of the child's body surface are classed as major.

Table 6.1 • Assessment of burned/scalded area as a percentage of total surface area

	0	1	5	10	15 years of age
A = ½ head	9½	8½	6½	5½	4½
B = ½ thigh	2¾	3¼	4	4½	4½
C = ½ lower leg	2½	2½	2¾	3	3¼

Thickness of burn

Treatment of the burned patient will depend not only on the extent of the injury but also on the depth of skin damaged. Thermal injuries are classified into superficial, partial thickness, full thickness, and deep dermal burns. Superficial burns are those with erythema only. The skin is bright red and painful. The burn heals well within a few days without scarring (for example sunburn). Partial thickness burns are those in which the top layer of skin has been destroyed but the dermis remains intact. The skin looks red and blisters will appear. Some blisters may be apparent immediately, but further blisters may develop over the next 24 hours. These are

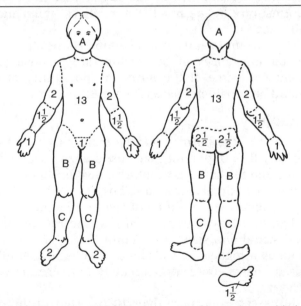

Fig 6.1 • Lund–Brouder chart for assessment of burned or scalded area.

painful. The wounds usually heal well in about two weeks. Full thickness burns are those in which the dermis has been destroyed. The dermis includes the layer of cells from which skin is formed, and contains hair follicles and nerve endings. As these are destroyed the wound will heal with scarring and will be painless. The burn usually looks white or black. The child may not appear to be in pain. These burns heal very slowly as they have to heal from the edges of the wound. Depending on the area involved and the size of the burn, these burns need skin grafting. Deep dermal burns occur where part of the dermis has been destroyed, leaving islands of skin cells. Burns which are deep dermal when seen initially may be converted to full thickness burns over a period of time as the residual cells may not survive owing to a poor blood supply or infection. Deep dermal burns are usually red, but blisters do not form easily. They are difficult to diagnose and initially should be treated as partial thickness burns. Skin grafting is usually done after a few days when further assessment of the burn takes place.

Site of burn

The site of the burn will influence the management of the child. Facial burns are serious, firstly because they indicate potential airway burns, and secondly because they may result in distressing scarring. Burns to the hands may cause problems, as scarring over joints can lead to contractures and damage to the skin of the fingers will lead to loss of sensation. Burns to the genitalia are difficult to manage and frequently become infected.

Intravenous infusion

If the burn covers more than 10 per cent of the body surface area, fluid replacement will be required and an intravenous infusion should be set up. The cannula can be inserted through burnt skin if an alternative suitable site cannot be found. The line can be used to give analgesia as well as fluid replacement. The child should be weighed so that fluid requirements and drug doses can be calculated accurately.

Other injuries

Particularly in burns from house fires or electrical burns,

additional trauma may be caused by the patient jumping or being thrown from a height. If the history of the injury or the circumstances in which the child was found suggest this, examination as described in Chapter 3 (major trauma) should be carried out. Special attention should be paid to head injury and cervical spine injury.

Major burns and scalds

- **Monitoring Investigations Treatment of the wound Indication for referral of burns or scalds**

All children whose burned or scalded area is 10 per cent or more of their total body surface are considered to have a major burn, however superficial the burn depth may appear. All these patients require intravenous colloid in addition to normal maintenance fluids. All burns, whatever their depth, are a cause of water, protein, and heat loss. *Senior help should be requested immediately.*

In the first four hours after the burn children with major burns should receive plasma, 5 per cent human albumin solution, or a colloid solution (for example Haemaccel) according to the following formula:

$$\text{plasma amount (ml)} = \frac{\% \text{ burn} \times \text{weight (kg)}}{2}$$

For example, for a 20 per cent burn in a 15 kg child 150 ml of plasma would be required.

This fluid should be infused over the first four hours after the accident. If there has been delay in bringing the patient to hospital the calculated amount should be given more rapidly so that the fluid is infused before the end of the first four hours following the injury.

In addition to this the patient's normal maintenance requirements should be given as 4 per cent dextrose with 0.18 per cent normal saline intravenously or, if the child is well enough, as oral drinks. Over the first four hours the maintenance fluid requirement will be 25 ml/kg.

Monitoring

1. Blood pressure, pulse, respiration rate, and mental status should be monitored at least hourly to observe for signs of circulatory collapse.

2. The urine output should be kept to at least 1 ml/kg/h and fluids and adjusted accordingly. The placement of a urinary catheter is almost always necessary to record urine output and keep the genital area 'clean'. (Keep a urine sample to be tested for specific gravity.)

3. Core temperature should be monitored.

Investigations

The following investigations should be made at presentation on all children with greater than 10 per cent burns.

1. Haemoglobin and haematocrit.

2. Blood group (cross-match for large burns).

3. Urea and electrolytes.

4. In patients who are shocked or who have respiratory problems from smoke inhalation (see p. 128), acid–base status and arterial oxygen concentration should be determined on an arterial sample.

5. Victims of smoke inhalation should have a baseline chest radiograph. This will usually be normal at first.

Treatment of the wound

The initial management of the major burn or scald prior to transfer to a burns unit is merely to clean with saline and cover in sterile sheets or clingfilm. If clothing is adhering to the wound, it should be carefully removed.

Indication for referral of burns or scalds

The following patients may need referral to a specialist burns or plastic surgery unit depending on the wound severity and the patient's individual circumstances.

1. All children with injuries covering more than 10 per cent of body surface area even if the burn appears to be only superficial.

2. Children who have been the victims of an electric shock.

3. Children who have been in a smoking fire and who have evidence of inhalation of smoke or fumes.

4. Full or suspected full thickness burns even if the area is small. These patients may require skin grafting, and so unless there are facilities for this procedure in the receiving hospital plastic surgery referral will be necessary. Early referral is important as modern treatment involves early grafting of burns.

5. Burns or scalds to the face, hands, perineum, or feet, even if they are less than 10 per cent may have poor cosmetic or functional outcome and, unless trivial, should be referred.

6. Patients in whom burns or scalds are one of multiple injuries will require transfer to a specialist unit. This unit must be able to treat all the child's injuries. The individual patient's injuries and local facilities will determine the most appropriate place for the child's management.

Inhalation injury

• **Management of inhalation injury**

In the initial stages, evidence of inhalation injury must be actively sought if suspected on history and clinical findings. Any patient who has suffered a burn in an enclosed space is a candidate for severe inhalation injury. Of course this includes all children who have been rescued from house fires. Signs which suggest inhalation injury include the following:

• burnt face
• evidence of burns in the mouth
• singed facial or nasal hairs
• hoarseness, wheezing, dyspnoea, or cough
• sputum with soot particles
• decreased level of consciousness.

These signs progress rapidly and frequent repeat observations are necessary.

Management of inhalation injury

1. *The anaesthetist should be called urgently.*
2. The patient should be given 100 per cent oxygen by mask.
3. In the event of wheezing or breathlessness nebulized salbutamol driven by oxygen may be helpful.
4. Intubation must be considered urgently. If intubation is delayed airway oedema may make the procedure impossible. A tracheostomy would then be necessary, and in patients with pulmonary damage and burn wounds a tracheostomy will predispose to severe pulmonary sepsis and a higher mortality.
5. Check arterial blood gases. (NB Pulse oximetry does not distinguish carboxyhaemoglobin from oxygenated haemoglobin). Measure carboxyhaemoglobin if possible.

Patients who are to be transferred to a specialist burns unit and are at risk from inhalation injury must be intubated before transfer. Patients with inhalation injury have fluid losses which exceed those of a simple skin burn. Fluid losses through the damaged tracheobronchial tree are difficult to estimate accurately, and pulmonary oedema is easily caused by fluid overload. Therefore these patients are difficult to manage and require careful circulatory monitoring in a burns intensive care unit.

Minor burns and scalds

• **Treatment of blisters Dressings Difficult areas**
Instructions to parents Follow-up

A child with burns that comprise less than 5 per cent of the surface area and are not full thickness can usually be managed as an out-patient. This will include the majority of children with burns and scalds attending an A & E department. Some children with burns of between 5 and 10 per cent of surface area would benefit from overnight observation and reassessment, but some can be treated as out-patients.

When the patient with a minor thermal injury arrives, the

first concern is analgesia. Cooling compresses and oral analgesics are usually sufficient, but some very distressed children
may need intramuscular morphine.

The wound should be cleansed with normal saline (no antiseptic need be used). The burn should then be dressed. There
are several different methods of dressing burns, and it is
necessary to become familiar with the accepted local practice.

Treatment of blisters

There are three alternative therapies for blisters: leave them
alone, drain them using a sterile needle, or completely deroof
them (i.e. cut away all the skin on top of the blister). Small
blisters and those on the hands and fingers may be left alone
or drained. Large blisters are uncomfortable and should be
drained or deroofed. When draining a blister, asepsis is important as infection may be introduced and the warm moist environment under the blister skin is an ideal incubation area.

Dressings

Paraffin gauze is an occlusive non-adhesive dressing which
will help to protect the burn. The dressing may be impregnated with chlorhexidine (Bactigras) or iodine (Inadine) to
help prevent infection. It is useful to put a few layers of dry
gauze on top to help stop any exudate soaking through. The
wound should then be covered with a dry bandage to keep the
gauze in place.

Silver sulphadiazine (Flamazine) cream helps to prevent
particular Gram-negative infections such as *Pseudomonas
aeruginosa*, but alters the appearance of the wound and makes
it more difficult to determine the depth of the burn.
Mupirocin (Bactroban) is effective against staphylococci (even
those that are resistant to methicillin); therefore it has a theo-
retical place in the management of burns to help prevent toxic
shock syndrome (p. 133). However, as yet there is no evidence
that it does so, and its widespread use may cause the development of resistant strains of staphylococci.

Difficult areas

Faces are difficult to dress and may be left exposed. Sometimes a colloid dressing is used. A layer of silver sulphadia-

zone or mupirocin can be applied to help prevent infection. Hands should not be put in tight dressings in which there is no finger movement or the fingers will become stiff. These burns may be dressed by applying a layer of cream and then putting the whole hand in a plastic bag. The burn is then covered but free movement is allowed. The arm should be elevated in a sling.

Instructions to parents

The dressing must be kept clean and dry. There is often exudate through the dressing when the burn is fresh, and if this is enough to soak the bandage, the child should be brought to the A & E department so that the external dressing can be changed. It must be made clear to parents that if the child becomes unwell or pyrexial or there is anxiety about the wound, he should be brought back immediately (see toxic shock syndrome (p. 133)).

Follow-up

The child should be reviewed after one or two days. The burn can be reassessed to check for areas of full thickness or deep dermal burn which may not have been apparent initially. Further blisters which have developed can be treated. The dressing is often soaked with exudate and can be changed. A new dressing should then be applied. The child can be reviewed again after a week. More frequent dressings are to be discouraged, as removing the dressing is painful and there is an increased risk of introducing infection.

Electrical burns

Electrical burns in the home are usually caused by children poking objects into electrical sockets or touching uninsulated wires. Older children can be injured through contact with high voltage wires, for example on railways.

Low voltage electrical injury causes arcing which produces discrete areas of full thickness burns (typically circular areas on the hand). There may be more than one area of burn (entry and exit points of current). Deeper structures may be damaged, and the area should be examined for blood vessel, nerve, and tendon damage. The injuries require surgical debridement and will often need grafting, particularly in areas of major function such as the hand.

The most severe injury is caused by transmission of electrical energy through the body. This produces an entry and exit wound. In high voltage electrical injury, the electricity disperses from the point of injury through the lowest pathway of resistance. This means that electrical injuries are usually much more serious and extensive internally than expected from examination of the skin which may merely show a superficial burn. The electrical shock often throws the child some distance, or the child may fall, so also look for associated injuries.

On admission, a patient who has suffered an electrical injury should generally be assessed for cardiopulmonary status, and shock or respiratory depression should be treated as appropriate. An ECG should be evaluated as there may be cardiac arrhythmias. The severity of the electrical injury is suggested by swelling and pain on passive extension of limbs, absence of pulse, or distal cyanosis and poor capillary refill.

These latter signs also suggest the development of compartment syndrome due to swelling from the electrical injury. Early decompression and even amputation is sometimes necessary. These patients must be urgently referred to a regional burns unit who will advise on immediate treatment and care during transfer.

More frequently, however, high voltage injury may arc around the surface of the victim, setting his clothes on fire and causing a direct flame injury without an internal electrical injury.

Chemical burns

Chemical burns are much less common in children than in adults. The burned area should always be sluiced with *large* amounts of water. No specific chemical antidotes should be used as the possible resultant heat of reaction will cause further skin injury. The resulting burn should be treated like any other burn or scald. A poisons centre should be consulted for further specific therapy. Occasionally inhalation of toxic vapours can produce secondary pulmonary injury. The management of this problem is similar to that of smoke inhalation injury.

Toxic shock syndrome

This condition is caused by a phage group 1 staphylococcal infection. It is uncommon, but can occur in burned and scalded patients or those with skin abrasions, whatever the size and depth of their injury. The clinical picture includes a high fever, headache, confusion, conjunctival and mucosal hyperaemia, scarlatiniform rash with secondary desquamation, subcutaneous oedema, vomiting, watery diarrhoea, hepatic and renal damage, disseminated intravascular coagulation, and severe prolonged shock.

Parents should be warned that if their child develops a fever, a rash, or diarrhoea, or becomes unwell, they should immediately bring him back to the A & E department.

Patients with toxic shock syndrome require intravenous colloid and anti-staphylococcal antibiotics such as flucloxacillin. *Urgent burns unit and paediatric help should be sought for management* and the patient may require transfer to an intensive care unit.

Sunburn

During the summer, large numbers of children attend A & E departments with sunburn. Young children and particularly infants can sustain serious burns to the skin after a relatively brief exposure to the sun.

Sunburn injuries should be assessed and treated as any other thermal injury.

Further reading

Muir, I. F. K., Barclay, T. L., and Settle, J. A. D. (1987). *Burns and their treatment* (3rd edn). Butterworths, London.

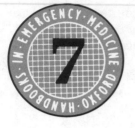

Poisoning

Poisoning

Suspected poisoning in children results in about 40 000 attendances at A & E departments per year in England and Wales. Less than half these children are admitted to hospital for treatment or observation.

Deaths are uncommon; there are usually less than 10 per year in England and Wales. The most common fatal poisons in children are the tricyclic antidepressants (TCAs).

The most frequently ingested drugs are analgesics (particularly paracetamol), anxiolytics, cough medicines, oral contraceptives, and dietary drugs such as vitamins. The most frequently ingested household products are bleaches, detergents, disinfectants, and petroleum distillates.

There has been a fall in the incidence of admissions for analgesic poisonings since the introduction of child-resistant containers for these drugs in the mid-1970s.

Types of poisoning incident

1. Accidental poisoning—this is the most common form of poisoning incident in childhood, and usually occurs in

134

children aged one to three years. The products involved are most commonly drugs, followed by household products, with a few children ingesting plants. Accidental poisoning usually occurs when the child is unsupervised. An increased incidence in poisoning is seen in households where there has been a recent disruption such as a new baby or a change of address, or where the mother is depressed.

2. Intentional overdose—suicide or para-suicide attempts are usually made by children in their teens.

3. Drug abuse—alcohol ingestion and solvent abuse are the most common forms of drug abuse in children in the UK.

4. Iatrogenic—the most common offender is diphenoxylate with atropine. This combination is toxic to some children at therapeutic doses. The most frequently fatal drug is digoxin.

5. Child abuse—rarely, symptoms are induced in children by their parents or caretakers by means of the administration of drugs. These incidents do not usually present as a poisoning incident but as an unknown illness (see Chapter 8).

General management of the poisoned child

• **History Examination General management**

History

Poisoned children usually present with a history of ingestion, but poisoning should be considered in any ill child, particularly any unconscious child, in whom the diagnosis is obscure. The poison container and its contents should be brought to hospital along with the child. Always assume the worst, i.e. if 10 tablets are missing assume that the child has taken them all. Children will ingest substances which are abhorrent to adults, for example bitter substances. Parents may not know or may be reluctant to admit how much of the poison their child has taken.

Points to note in the history are as follows:

- which poisons have been taken?
- an estimate of how much has been taken (examine the container);
- at what time ingestion occurred;
- description of any subsequent symptoms;
- any acute or chronic illness and any current medication.

Examination

Frequently the child shows no immediate ill-effects from the poisoning. Sometimes evidence of the substance involved may be apparent, for example the small of a domestic substance on the child's clothes, or coloured particles, or burns in the mouth. Many drugs produce characteristic signs (Table 7.1).

General management

1. Resuscitation—if necessary this should follow the usual procedures (see Chapter 2).
2. Airway care—if the conscious level is depressed intubation should be considered, particularly if gastric lavage is to be

Table 7.1 • Specific signs of drug overdose

Pinpoint pupils	Opiates
Dilated pupiles	Atropine (more commonly, atropine-containing compounds, e.g. diphenoxylate/atropine), TCAs
Drowsiness	Alcohol, sedatives, narcotics, hypnotics, diphenoxylate/atropine, aspirin, TCAs
Confusion, ataxia, excitability	Alcohol, TCAs, antihistamines, salbutamol, dexamphetamine, solvent abuse
Convulsions	Alcohol, dexamphetamine, TCAs, theophylline, lithium
Extrapyramidal dystonic reactions	phenothiazines (e.g. prochlorperazine), metoclopramide
Cardiac arrhythmias	TCAs, amphetamines, potassium, theophylline, salbutamol, digoxin, beta-blockers
Hyperventilation	Salicylates
Hypotension	Sedatives, narcotics, hypnotics, iron
Hypertension plus tachycardia	Amphetamines, sympathomimetics
Haematemesis	Iron, salicylates

Box 7.1 **Points to note on examination of poisoned child**

- Conscious level
- blood pressure and pulse rate
- Respiratory rate and depth
- Pupil size and reactivity
- Skin and mouth for contact burns

performed. The anaesthetist should use a cuffed endotracheal tube in older unconscious children when gastric lavage is performed.

3. Respiration—ventilate if respiration is inadequate. A pulse oximeter is helpful. If the patient is unconscious or there is any concern about respiratory adequacy, arterial blood gas should be estimated.

4. Hypotension—if there is hypotension insert an intravenous cannula and give aliquots of a plasma expander at 10 ml/kg in addition to elevating the foot of the trolley. Monitor ECG.

5. Keep the patient warm—some drugs may cause hypothermia.

6. Check blood glucose levels in any unconscious patient—consider a trial of naloxone (10 µg/kg intravenously initially).

Elimination of the poison

- **Activated charcoal Recommendations for management Admission**

Many children do not need stomach evacuation as they have not taken anything dangerous. There is continuing controversy about the best way to empty the stomach of ingested poisons. There are two main methods of doing this: gastric lavage or induced emesis using ipecacuanha. With either method, even under ideal conditions, less than half the poison is retrieved.

Problems with lavage include the unpleasantness of the procedure, a small risk of accidental perforation of the oesophagus, and a risk of aspiration of gastric contents. Lavage may wash poisons into the duodenum and enhance absorption. The limitations of gastric lavage in children are largely due to the small diameter of tube which can be used. Many pills are too large to pass through a narrow tube. However, lavage may sometimes be useful through its mechanical action in breaking up concretions of pills, such as insoluble aspirin and iron, in the stomach. The fluid for gastric lavage should be one-fifth normal saline in 4 per cent dextrose (except in special circumstances; see individual poisons), and aliquots of 10 ml/kg should be used. In older children water can be used. The stomach should first be aspirated and then lavage should be carried out with the patient in the left Trendelenburg position. A sample of the stomach aspirate should be saved for chemical analysis if necessary.

Emesis induced by ipecacuanha is safer and more efficacious than gastric lavage in the vast majority of poisoning incidents, with the exception of patients with a depressed conscious level. The time from administration of ipecacuanha to emesis is usually about 20 minutes, and during this time the child must not lie down. Occasionally vomiting may persist for several hours. The dose of ipecacuanha for children over one year is 15 ml. Over seven years of age 30 ml can be used. This should be followed by a drink of 100–200 ml of water or fruit juice (seek paediatric advice in infants—dose of ipecacuanha is 10 ml). A second dose may be given if vomiting has not occurred within 20 minutes.

Never evacuate the stomach, by any means, after the ingestion of corrosive substances. It is usual not to evacuate the stomach after ingestion of paraffin, petroleum products, turpentine, etc. because of the risk of inhalation pneumonitis. However, evacuation may occasionally be recommended after the ingestion of very large amounts of petroleum products. Seek advice from a poisons centre.

If saline has been given at home, as an emetic, by the parent, the patient may be hypernatraemic—check the serum sodium.

Activated charcoal

Activated charcoal absorbs some toxic substances, particularly those that are weakly acidic. It is useful for the treatment of poisoning with TCAs, theophylline, digoxin, barbiturates, salicylate, and carbamazepine, and will increase the non-renal elimination of these drugs when given in repeated doses over 48 hours. This latter activity is thought to act by binding the drug in the bowel, thus allowing it to diffuse from the blood into the bowel lumen where it can in turn be bound to the charcoal.

Charcoal is at its most effective if given very soon after ingestion of the poison. Patient acceptability is low, as a large volume of the black gritty liquid needs to be taken. There is a particular problem in giving activated charcoal to a patient in whom emesis has been induced by the use of ipecacuanha. If the charcoal is given first, the emetic will not work as it will be bound to the charcoal. If the emetic is given first, the charcoal is often vomited. Therefore there is a case for stomach evacuation by gastric lavage if activated charcoal is to be used subsequently. A further advantage is that the charcoal can be introduced via the gastric tube. there is some evidence that charcoal alone, without gastric evacuation, may be effective treatment for poisonings.

Recommendations for management

1. Many household products (most cosmetics, paints, and inks) and some drugs (most antibiotics, vitamins, and the contraceptive pill) are not toxic and do not require gastric evacuation or patient observation. If in doubt ask for advice from a poisons centre.

2. Emesis induced by ipecacuanha is indicated for poisonings with potentially toxic tablets/capsules, especially those within the previous one to two hours.

3. Gastric lavage is indicated under the following conditions:
   - in association with endotracheal intubation in an unconscious patient (seek anaesthetic help);
   - in patients who cannot be persuaded to take ipecacuanha or who have failed to vomit after two doses of ipecacuanha, and gastric emptying is thought essential;
   - in paraquat poisoning, after lavage a slurry of Fuller's earth can be passed down the tube to bind any unabsorbed paraquat (keep a sample of the gastric contents to test with dithionite for the presence of paraquat);

- in patients who have taken large doses of insoluble aspirin or iron tablets to attempt to break up the concretions in the stomach, and to give sodium bicarbonate or a specific antidote (see pp. 137 and 146).

4. Activated charcoal is currently advised for many poisons, especially liquid drugs. It is particularly indicated for the treatment of poisonings with TCAs, theophylline, digoxin and barbiturates. The dose is 1–2 g/kg. It may require administration by nasogastric tube or syringe, as patient acceptability is often poor.

Admission

Many children require observation for 12–24 hours. Some children may be discharged after observation for 4–6 hours if the drugs that they have taken will have passed their peak serum levels by that time.

Box 7.2 **Criteria for admission of poisoned patient**

- symptomatic patient
- potentially toxic ingestion
- history unclear

Prevention of poisoning incidents

1. When the child is discharged a discussion should be held with the parents about the need for prevention of further incidents. A lockable medicine cabinet should be recommended, and advice given on the safe disposal of old unwanted medicines.
2. Child-resistant containers have proved a great success in reducing the number of admissions to hospital of children with analgesic poisoning. These containers should be used for all drugs and household products wherever possible.
3. The parents should be warned against transferring drugs or household products to unlabelled bottles.
4. It is helpful if the health visitor visits the home after a poisoning incident for further discussion on prevention.

Poison information services

It is often difficult to assess the potential toxicity of the wide variety of substances that may be ingested. It is also useful to check the up-to-date treatment of common poisons. Poison information centres have been set up to collate information about poisons and can give details on identification and treatment. The two main centres are the National Poisons Information Service at New Cross Hospital, London, telephone number 071–635—9191 and the Scottish Poisons Information Bureau at Edinburgh, telephone number 031–229–2477. The Poisons Information Service provides a 24 hour service.

Specific drug poisoning

- **Paracetamol Salicylates and aspirin Narcotic analgesics Tricyclic antidepressants Benzodiazepines Iron poisoning Phenothiazines Digoxin**

Paracetamol

An excess of paracetamol is extremely toxic, but children are more resistant than adults to its effect. The toxic dose for adults is 150–250 mg/kg. The toddler who takes some extra paracetamol elixir is rarely severely poisoned, but the adolescent who takes over 20 tablets is at serious risk of liver damage without treatment with acetylcysteine. Initially there may be no clinical features of toxicity, but later the patient may develop nausea, vomiting, upper abdominal pain, and tenderness. Finally the patient may develop acute liver failure, and a small percentage develop renal failure.

Management

1. Emesis should be induced by giving ipecacuanha up to four hours after ingestion.
2. Measure serum paracetamol level at four hours.
3. Assess toxicity risk on the basis of this level.
4. Administer acetylcysteine intravenously if the paracetamol levels are above 200 mg/l (1320 µmol/l) at four hours. If the

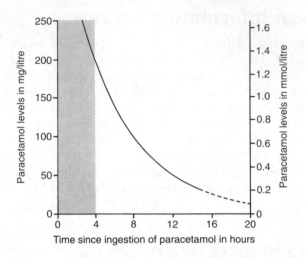

Fig 7.1 • Graph to estimate need for acetylcysteine treatment in paracetamol poisoning

patient presents later than four hours Fig. 7.1 indicates the paracetamol level above which treatment is required. A dose of 150 mg/kg acetylcysteine over 15 minutes initially followed by an infusion of 50 mg/kg over four hours should be given. Acetylcysteine occasionally causes a rash. Bronchospasm may occur in asthmatics, and anaphylaxis has been reported.

Note: Acetylcysteine is most efficient if started within eight hours of the overdose, but can be started at up to 15 hours.

If the patient presents at more than 15 hours, discuss the management with a poisons centre. If the result will not be known until more than eight hours after ingestion, oral methionine can be used in non-vomiting patients suspected of significant overdose prior to receipt of the paracetamol level result.

Admission This depends on the paracetamol level. If the level is clearly below the toxic level (see Fig. 7.1), the child can be sent home; otherwise admission and treatment are necessary. Patients who present with a history of a possible large overdose, however long after ingestion, should be admitted for monitoring and, if necessary, treatment of hepatic or renal failure. Children will usually need admission for psychiatric and social reasons.

Salicylates and aspirin

Aspirin poisoning is less common than paracetamol poisoning. Children's preparations of aspirin are less readily available as they are discouraged in children under 12 years of age (owing to the possible association with Reye's syndrome). It is important to remember the high salicylate content of oil of wintergreen. The threshold for salicylate toxicity is close to that of therapeutic levels, and children are very susceptible to toxicity.

Clinical features of aspirin poisoning in children are often different to those in adults. Children frequently develop a metabolic acidosis and hypoglycaemia. Loss of consciousness is rare but implies severe poisoning. Common features are nausea and vomiting, deafness or tinnitus, sweating, hyperventilation, vasodilatation, and tachycardia. Convulsions occasionally occur.

Management

1. If the overdose was small and/or a soluble preparation emesis may be induced by ipecacuanha.

2. If the overdose was large and of an insoluble preparation gastric lavage with 1 per cent sodium bicarbonate solution or water is indicated.

3. If the overdose was very recent, i.e. less than one hour, activated charcoal should be left in the stomach.

4. The serum salicylate level and blood sugar levels should be measured at two hours. Salicylate levels of less than 250 mg/l are unlikely to be associated with symptoms.

5. A symptomatic child, or one with a salicylate level of more than 500 mg/l, should be treated with an intravenous infusion of one-fifth normal saline and 4 per cent dextrose. Blood sugar levels should be measured at regular intervals, and the child should be referred immediately to the paediatricians as forced alkaline diuresis may be required in some instances.

6. Children with salicylate levels of 250 mg/l or more should be admitted for observation, as levels may rise.

Narcotic analgesics

The clinical features of poisoning are similar even with different types of opiates. The main cause for concern is respiratory depression which may occur quite late after the poisoning. The child may become comatose and have convulsions, hypotension, and arrhythmias.

Pinpoint pupils are an important diagnostic sign but are not always present.

Management

1. Ensure an adequate airway and prevent aspiration of vomit by lateral positioning.
2. Ventilate with bag and mask if necessary. Anaesthetic help should be sought urgently if there is respiratory depression.
3. Assess conscious level.
4. Administer intravenous naloxone (dose 0.2 mg for a child less than one-year old, 0.4 mg for a child 1–12 years old, 0.8 mg for a child over 12 years of age) if the child is symptomatic. Naloxone has a short half-life and this dose may need to be repeated every 15–20 minutes. Sometimes larger doses or an infusion are needed.
5. Treat by emesis or lavage depending on conscious level.
6. Children should be admitted and observed carefully as depression of conscious level and respiration may occur suddenly.

Tricyclic antidepressants

These are extremely toxic compounds and the most common cause of death in childhood poisonings. TCAs are prescribed for children with enuresis (but are ineffectual) and are widely prescribed for adults. TCAs block the uptake of monoamines in the brain and also have anticholinergic effects. They have a direct effect on cell membranes and this accounts for their cardiotoxicity.

Symptoms appear within four hours of overdose and include dry mouth, blurred vision, drowsiness, and tachycardia.

This may progress to coma, convulsions, respiratory depression, hypotension, and cardiac arrhythmias.

Management

1. Institute continuous ECG monitoring.

2. Evacuate stomach. Gastric lavage with airway protection is necessary if the patient is drowsy or comatose. Gastric lavage is preferable to emesis with ipecacuanha if activated charcoal is to be left in the stomach after evacuation.

3. Give activated charcoal (1–2 g/kg).

4. All children must be admitted for ECG monitoring and many will need intensive care monitoring. A wide QRS complex indicates serious toxicity. Adequate oxygenation and avoidance of acidosis are vital in order to decrease the risk of arrhythmias. An arterial blood gas estimation should be done. If bradycardia or arrhythmias develop, the child is probably hypoxic and needs ventilating. If arrhythmias persist, despite ventilation on oxygen, give sodium bicarbonate 1 mmol/kg intravenously. This alters the protein binding of the TCA and reduces the free drug concentration and the cardiotoxicity. Urgent specialist cardiology and poisons advice should be sought in the event of arrhythmias.

5. Treat convulsions with diazepam intravenously. Artificial ventilation will probably also be required in this instance.

Benzodiazepines

The ready availability of these drugs makes them a common cause of poisoning. They are relatively safe, with the main effect being CNS depression. The child will appear drowsy and may be ataxic. In more serious overdoses coma and hypotension can occur occasionally.

Management

• Induce emesis with ipecacuanha unless drowsy.
• Admit the child for observation.

Iron poisoning

This commonly available substance is extremely poisonous, causing severe gastric haemorrhage and shock. The initial symptoms are nausea, vomiting, abdominal pain, and diarrhoea.

Management

1. If the patient is symptomatic on arrival, intramuscular desferrioxamine (30 mg/kg) should be given immediately (take care that this does not enter a vein as rapid infusion of desferrioxamine may cause anaphylaxis).

2. Gastric lavage should be performed with airway protection if the child is drowsy. The lavage fluid should be 1 per cent sodium bicarbonate and 5–10g of desferrioxamine should be left in the stomach.

3. The child should have an intravenous infusion sited, and depending on symptomatology may need the infusion of desferrioxamine over the next 24 hours. Advice from a poisons centre should be sought.

4. In cases of large overdose an abdominal radiograph after gastric evacuation will help in determining how much iron is left in the bowel.

5. All cases should be admitted to paediatric care and some will need intensive care.

Phenothiazines

The main side-effects of phenothiazine poisoning in children are drowsiness and extrapyramidal symptoms.

Management

1. Emesis should be induced or lavage performed with airway protection if the patient is drowsy.

2. In cases of a large overdose activated charcoal may be helpful.

3. Extrapyramidal side-effects should be treated with benzotropine.

Digoxin

Overdose is more common in hospital than at home. Emesis or lavage should be followed by the use of activated charcoal. Cardiac monitoring is essential. Digibind (digoxin-specific antibody fragments) can be infused as a specific antidote in severe poisoning. Poisons centre advice should be sought urgently.

Household products poisoning

- Caustic soda   Methyl alcohol and ethylene glycol (antifreeze)   Ethyl alcohol

Toxic household products include bleaches, detergents, disinfectants, caustics, and compounds containing petroleum distillates. Most children swallow very small amounts of these products owing to their unpleasant taste, but often spill a lot. Therefore morbidity is low. However, it is important that each case is investigated thoroughly. More than one substance may have been ingested, and it is often surprising how toxic some apparently innocent substances are. Usually the advice of a poisons centre is needed in the case of proprietary products whose constituents are not clear.

In most cases emetics should not be given. Substances such as detergents and bleaches can cause chemical burns to the sensitive oesophageal mucosa which would be worsened by emesis. Petroleum distillates carry a high risk of pneumonitis and pulmonary oedema if aspirated, and therefore emesis is contra-indicated. Milk should be given to help dilute the poison and further treatment given as recommended by a poisons centre.

Caustic soda

Caustic soda is used as a cleaning agent and is found in dishwasher powders. Even a small amount can cause a stricture of the oesophagus. Milk should be given, and all children who have ingested alkalis should be admitted and referred to the surgeon in case oesophagoscopy is required.

Methyl alcohol and ethylene glycol (antifreeze)

Ingestion of these two substances is relatively uncommon in children. The patient appears inebriated but there is no smell of alcohol. Rapid recognition of these poisons is important as there is a specific antidote, i.e. ethyl alcohol. The poisons centre should be contacted for detailed advice.

Ethyl alcohol

Children of all ages ingest alcohol. Younger children take it as an accidental ingestion either as an alcoholic beverage or by consuming cosmetics containing alcohol. Only small amounts of alcohol are necessary to produce symptoms in childhood, and children easily develop hypoglycaemia with alcohol poisoning.

The clinical features are similar to those in adults, and if the patient is unconscious, care must be taken to prevent the aspiration of vomit. The blood sugar level must be measured and an intravenous dextrose infusion set up if the patient is significantly intoxicated or is hypoglycaemic. Make sure that there is no other cause for the patient's condition which may be associated with alcohol intake, such as drugs, trauma, or illness. Patients need observation until they are fully conscious and mobile. Treatment aimed at speeding up the elimination of the alcohol, i.e. lavage, intravenous fructose, and intravenous naloxone are ineffective and unnecessary. Frequent episodes of alcoholic intoxication in teenagers may indicate psychiatric or social problems and should lead to psychiatric referral.

Ingested foreign bodies

• **Button batteries**

Rounded non-penetrating foreign bodies are the most common objects swallowed. Of these, coins feature most frequently. Once past the pylorus, foreign bodies will pass through the bowel uneventfully. Removal is usually only indicated for those that stick in the oesophagus.

Children who have ingested a radio-opaque foreign body, such as a coin, should have a radiograph of the neck, chest, and upper abdomen with genital protection. If the object is in the pharynx or oesophagus, the child should be referred for its removal at oesophagoscopy. Most of these children will be symptomatic with dysphagia, dyspnoea, dysphonia, or retrosternal pain, but some will be symptom free.

If the object has passed into the stomach or bowel, the child may be allowed home and the parents told to search the stools until the object is found. If it has not been found after two weeks, then the child should return for a further X-ray, and surgical referral arranged for those in whom the foreign body is still visible. In the meantime the parents should be instructed to bring the child back to hospital if he should develop abdominal pain or vomiting, or pass blood per rectum.

Ingested sharp objects, such as an open safety-pin or pointed nail, should result in an immediate surgical referral as the child will require observation. Surprisingly, most of these objects pass through the bowel leaving the mucosa unscathed. The necessity for surgical removal is low.

Button batteries

Small button batteries are easily swallowed by children. A few may disintegrate in the bowel causing secondary problems. The type of battery which has been ingested should be identified. The most dangerous are new mercury batteries. The child should have a radiograph of the neck, chest, and upper abdomen with genital protection, and if the battery is in the oesophagus it should be removed at oesophagoscopy. The management of batteries in the stomach is debatable, and specialist advice should be sought from a poisons centre as to whether the child should be observed or the batteries removed.

Suicide attempts

Toddlers take poisons accidentally. However, in the older child the overdose is most likely to be deliberate. The overdose is most commonly a 'cry for help'. Unfortunately, some of these children may succeed in killing themselves. The overdose may also be an indication of an underlying psychiatric illness.

In all cases the poisoning needs to be dealt with in the usual manner. It is them important that the child and parents be interviewed, usually by a psychiatrist experienced in adolescent problems. No child who has intentionally taken a poison should be discharged without psychiatric assessment and follow-up.

Substance abuse

- Management

Solvent and drug abuse is becoming more common in children—some even as young as seven years of age. Many solvents are readily available and include glue, chlorinated hydrocarbons (found in cleaning fluids, paints, varnishes, lacquers, and dyes), fluorocarbons (used as aerosol propellants and in fire extinguishers), petrol, acetones, butane, propane, etc. Abuse may lead to death caused directly by the toxicity of the substance or from trauma, anoxia, or aspiration of gastric contents during intoxication. Clinically, the patient may have similar symptoms to those caused by alcohol intoxication, including euphoria, blurred vision, tinnitus, slurred speech, ataxia, headache, abdominal pain, nausea, vomiting, chest pain, and bronchospasm. More serious effects include convulsions, respiratory depression, coma, and cardiac arrhythmias. Signs of a rash around the mouth and nose and suggestive of chronic solvent abuse.

Management

Stopping the inhalation will relieve the intoxication and no specific treatment is needed, except for complications such as convulsions or respiratory depression. The patient should be referred to the psychiatric department for further management.

Ingestion of plants

Berries are the most common plant parts to be ingested and the most likely to be poisonous. Emesis induced by ipecacuanha and observation for 6–12 hours is recommended for ingestion of unknown berries.

Laburnum seeds are one of the most common types of plant material ingested. Most children are asymptomatic. Vomiting, drowsiness, abdominal pain, mucosal irritation, and hypersalivation may occur, but serious poisoning is very rare. Emesis and observation are the treatment requirements if more than a few seeds have been ingested.

Yew berries cause gastrointestinal symptoms, tachycardia, and then bradycardia and hypotension. Children should be treated with ipecacuanha and observation.

Holly and honeysuckle seeds produce gastrointestinal symptoms, and emesis should be produced for the ingestion of more than a few berries. Arum lily (cuckoo-pint, lords and ladies) and *Dieffenbachia* sp. (Leopard lily) seeds cause buccal and pharyngeal pain and swelling. Cold drinks should be offered and the child observed for several hours.

The common berries berberis, cotoneaster, mahonia, pyracanthus, and rowan are non-toxic, but a mild gastro-intestinal upset may occur.

Poisons centre advice should be sought for ingestions of unknown plants and in cases of doubt.

Further reading

1. Proudfoot, A. T. (1982). *Diagnosis and management of acute poisoning.* Blackwell Scientific, Oxford.
2. Vale, J. A. and Meredith, T. J. (ed.) (1981). *Poisoning: diagnosis and treatment.* Update Books, London.
3. Craft, A. W. (1988). Accidental poisoning. *Archives of Disease in Childhood,* **63,** 584–6.
4. Sibert, J. R. and Routledge, P. A. (1991). Accidental poisoning in children: can we admit fewer children with safety? *Archives of Disease in Childhood,* **66,** 263–6.

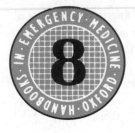

Child abuse

Key points in child abuse

1 If abuse is suspected, ask for a senior paediatric opinion.

2 Particularly consider the possibility of abuse when examining injured babies of less than one year of age.

3 In a child with suspected sexual abuse, genital examination constitutes further abuse and should be undertaken by one experienced doctor only unless life-threatening bleeding requires immediate aid.

Child abuse

The management of suspected child abuse should be directed to the following:

• treat the child's injuries, including the psychological ones
• cooperate with others to ensure the child's safety.

Aetiology

1. Abuse is more common in a family where one or both parents suffered abuse themselves in childhood.

2. Abuse is more frequently identified in the children of younger parents living in stressful social conditions, but the problem can be found throughout society.

3. Children under five years of age are more usually victims of abuse than are older children, and those under two years of age are most at risk from permanent injury or death.

4. Abuse of older children is usually associated more with control and over-harsh chastisement than stemming from an attachment problem as in abuse of younger children.

Recognition of abuse in the A & E department

• **Types of abuse   Physical abuse   Physical features of non-accidental injury**

The experienced A & E doctor is in a good position to recognize abuse as he will have had the opportunity to see a large number of accidental injuries and therefore will be familiar with the types of injury that children incur accidentally and the history that usually accompanies that injury.

Box 8.1

It is important to be clear that it is not the duty of the A & E senior house officer to diagnose child abuse. His duty is to recognize possible abuse and to refer these children for a senior paediatric opinion.

The A & E senior house officer must remember that in referring to a patient with an injury about whose origin he is doubtful, he is not accusing a parent of abuse. He is merely asking a more experienced colleague for an opinion on a difficult case. A non-accusatory approach is vital—worries about abuse may be unfounded and if the concerns are realized, antagonism is unprofitable.

Child abuse may be recognized by certain characteristics of the child, the history of the injury, and the injury itself. The suspicion of abuse is usually based on a combination of historical and physical features.

Types of abuse

More than one form of abuse may coexist in individual children; for example a sexually abused child may also be physically injured. A physically injured child may also suffer emotional deprivation, sometimes leading to failure to thrive.

8.2 Types of abuse

1. Physical abuse
   (non-accidental injury)
   • superficial lesions—bruises, abrasions, lacerations
   • bone injuries
   • internal injuries—intracranial and visceral
   • burns and scalds
2. Sexual abuse
3. Neglect (psychosocial deprivation)
4. Non-accidental poisoning
5. Suffocation
6. Munchausen syndrome by proxy

Physical abuse

Features in the history of the injury which should alert the doctor

1. Inappropriate delay in seeking advice after a significant injury, for example a bad fracture or burn. (*Note*: prompt A & E attendance for injury does not rule out abuse.)
2. Previous history of frequent accidents to the child.
3. The history of the injury is inconsistent with the findings on physical examination.
4. Absence of a reasonable explanation of the injury when one would normally expect one.
5. No history of accident given, but the child presented as 'crying' or 'not walking' with a significant injury present.
6. Significantly different explanations have been given for the same injuries.

7. The child is said to have contributed to his injury in a way which is inconsistent with his development.

8. Another child is said to have caused the injury in a way that is inconsistent with that child's development.

9. The adult may appear less concerned than most parents about the child's injury or may become hostile when the history is sought.

10. The child's explanation may differ from the adult's. If he is old enough, always ask the child what happened.

General examination of a child in whom there is concern about abuse

1. It is important to examine thoroughly any child in whom there is a concern about non-accidental injury (NAI) in order to look for other signs of injury. All clothing should be removed, although this may be done in stages so as not to distress the child.

2. General demeanour—the child may be unusually quiet, although the classic 'frozen watchfulness' of the frequently injured child is rare and many children are very affectionate and clinging to their abusers. An indiscriminate friendliness to strangers is sometimes a feature of abused children and, if noted, should be recorded.

3. Assessment of the growth status is important. The child should be weighed and measured, and the results plotted on growth charts. Non-organic failure to thrive is sometimes associated with physical abuse.

Physical features of non-accidental injury

Some findings, in injured children such as retinal haemorrhage and fractured ribs, are highly suggestive of NAI. Others are sufficient to alert the doctor to the need for further consultation, such as bruising to a baby's face or a fracture in a child aged under one year.

Soft tissue injuries which are suggestive of NAI

1. Fingertip bruising—several small round bruises grouped together, perhaps on either side of cheeks or around a limb.

2. Slap marks—groups of linear bruises arising where a hard blow from a hand has forced blood out of adjoining skin

capillaries, forming lines on either side of the hand or fingers impression. This bruising is often across the face, legs, or buttocks.

3. Bruising on both sides of, or inside, the pinna—this injury is not common accidentally.

4. Bruises showing the pattern of the artefact which caused them. This will be a line of bruising on either side of the object's impression, for example belt or stick marks.

5. Bruising of various ages, as shown by a change of colour from purplish red to yellow, suggests injuries at different times.

6. Any bruising in a non-mobile baby.

7. Torn frenulum—this may be caused by the thrusting of a bottle into a baby's mouth, but it does sometimes occur accidentally.

8. Bite marks—clearly, human bite marks are intentional, but it is not always easy to determine whether they are of adult or child origin. A dentist's opinion is most helpful.

Common patterns of accidental bruising

- Forehead in toddlers
- Knees and shins in any ambulant child.
- Front of hips, outer thighs, and forearms in school-age children.
- Overlying spinous processes in school-age children.

Scratches on babies' faces are usually self-inflicted. In older children many other bruises, such as black eyes and buttock bruises, may be either accidental or non-accidental and need to be considered in the light of the history and complete examination. All mobile children have some accidental bruises, and some children have many.

Fractures Most accidental fractures occur in children of school age. Extra consideration of the possibility of abuse should be given to fractures in children who are under two years of age and particularly in those under one year of age. A single fracture in a child aged under two years is usually an accidental injury, but if it is accompanied by signs such as multiple bruises, or failure to thrive, or an inconsistent history, then referral for a senior opinion should be made.

Features of possible non-accidental fractures

1. Rib fractures are usually found incidentally on a chest radiograph and are identified by callus that forms 7–10 days after injury. Rib fractures rarely occur accidentally, except for example in a severe road traffic accident. Inflicted rib fractures are usually posterior.

2. Multiple metaphyseal and epiphyseal fractures can be caused when a child is pulled, twisted, or shaken by the limbs or trunk. The delicate growing areas of bone are damaged by pulling and shearing forces.

3. Multiple fractures in different stages of healing are highly suggestive of abuse in the absence of bone disease.

4. Spiral fractures of a long bone are more common than transverse fractures in abuse, but both may occur in either accidental or non-accidental injury.

5. Any fracture in a non-mobile baby.

6. Children may be presented as crying, limping, or refusing to walk with no history of injury given by the parent.

7. The injury may have been presented late, often again with no history of injury.

8. The finding of new periosteal bone on a radiograph indicates sub-periosteal damage some 10–14 days previously. This may be associated with a fracture or may occur alone from a limb injury.

Head injuries Head injury is the most common cause of death from trauma. In the school-age child the main cause of head injury is the road traffic accident. In the first year of life most serious intracranial injuries result from abuse. All non-mobile babies presenting with a head injury should have a skull X-ray. Although the history may be of a trivial injury, it may be false. Accidental head injury in a non-mobile baby usually occurs when the infant is dropped or falls, for example from a work surface onto a hard floor.

Severe intracranial haemorrhage, usually without skull fracture, may be caused in an infant who is violently shaken. The baby may be presented as generally unwell, drowsy, apnoeic, or convulsing. Retinal haemorrhage is characteristic of this injury.

Characteristics of accidental skull fracture in infants
• Single linear fracture or small depressed fracture.
• Commonly in parietal bone.

Characteristics of non-accidental skull fracture
• Multiple wide branching fractures.
• More than one skull bone is involved, and fracture of the occiput is particularly characteristic.
• Underlying brain damage is more common.

Abdominal injuries A few children have serious intra-abdominal injuries which may be life-threatening. Presentation is usually as an ill or shocked child, or one with abdominal pain, distension, or rectal bleeding. Splenic or hepatic damage or rupture of the duodenum or small bowel may occur following severe blows to the abdomen. The management should be as indicated for severe abdominal trauma (see Chapter 3), but note should be taken of any associated bruising or other physical features.

Non-accidental burns and scalds Estimates of the incidence of non-accidental burns and scalds vary from 1 to 16 per cent of all children presenting at hospital with thermal injury.

Accidental scalding usually leaves splash marks, and the most common injury is the scalded face and chest of the toddler who pulls a hot liquid down over himself. Accidental contact burns commonly affect the palms of the hands, the knuckles, and the forearms.

Characteristics of non-accidental burns and scalds
1. Glove or stocking scalds which are caused by forced immersion in too hot water.
2. Some buttock and perineal burns.
3. Sometimes the imprint of a hot object may be seen on the skin at a site where the child could not have easily touched the object accidentally, for example the abdomen.
4. Cigarette burns, particularly if more than one. Cigarette burns are circular, deep, and have a raised indurated edge.

The differential diagnosis of physical abuse

- Conditions in which pathological bruising may mimic non-accidental injury   Conditions in which skin lesions may mimic burns   Conditions in which bone disease may mimic non-accidental fractures

Although physical abuse is probably underdiagnosed, it is also sometimes over-diagnosed. A clotting screen and full blood count should identify patients who have a clotting disorder accounting for their bruising. A skeletal survey which is performed to look for old fractures in a child suspected of being abused is also useful in identifying bone disease. These investigations would normally be ordered by the paediatrician after referral and assessment.

Conditions in which pathological bruising may mimic non-accidental injury

- Henoch–Schonlein purpura.
- Idiopathic thrombocytopenic purpura.
- Leukaemia.
- Clotting disorders such as haemophilia.
- Drug-induced thrombocytopenia, for example sulphonamides.
- Rare connective tissue disorders such as Ehlers–Danlos syndrome

In addition, the commonly seen 'Mongolian blue spot' may be mistaken for bruising. This is a congenital skin lesion of no clinical significance. It is slatey-blue in colour and usually occurs on the lower back (although it may be found at any site). It is usually found in non-Caucasian children, although it can occasionally be seen in Caucasian children.

Conditions in which skin lesions may mimic burns

1. Impetigo is sometimes mistaken for cigarette burns. The cigarette burn is an ulcerated lesion with a raised rim.
2. Staphyloccocal skin infection in infants may resemble scalds, but in either case such an infant would require admission.

Conditions in which bone disease may mimic non-accidental fractures

- Osteogenesis imperfecta.
- Rickets.
- Pathological fracture through tumour or cyst.
- Copper deficiency.
- Caffey's disease.

All these bone diseases are uncommon.

Management of suspected physical abuse

The suspicion of NAI usually arises from a combination of historical and physical features of an injury or of concern about a child, and rarely from one pathognomonic sign. The duty of the A & E senior house officer is to refer for senior opinion any patient with an injury about whose origin he feels concerned. The decision whether to tell the parent that the referral is about the possibility of abuse is difficult. It is reasonable merely to say, 'I would like another opinion'. If the child is removed by the parent before the paediatrician arrives, the problem should be discussed with him and the social worker.

The suspicion that child abuse has occurred may be the first stage in a long process of investigation, protection, and re-habilitation that involves teamwork between several agencies including the medical profession, social work departments, and the police. In most areas police departments have a specialist team of police officers, both male and female, who are trained and experienced in child protection work.

Social workers have a statutory duty to protect children, and the social services department must be informed of all suspected cases of abuse. In the UK social workers can seek legal orders from a magistrate, including an Emergency Protection Order, and may carry out a Supervision Order.

Finally, it is imperative that all historical and physical findings in a case of suspected child abuse should be carefully documented in contemporaneously written notes. Bruises or other lesions should be described in words and also measured and drawn on a diagram. Where possible, a photograph of the injury is an invaluable record.

Sexual abuse

- **Management of child presenting with acute perineal injury (straddle injury) Management of child presented as having been raped Presentation of chronic child sexual abuse**

The incidence of child sexual abuse is unknown. It ranges from exposure of the child to pornographic information to penetrative rape. Boys and girls of all ages may be affected. The abuser is usually a male relative, cohabitant, or neighbour.

As far as the A & E department is concerned, sexual abuse may present in three broad ways.

1. As an acute event, usually presenting as perineal injury and occasionally as clear rape.

2. With parental anxiety on first suspicion of sexual abuse.

3. As a more chronic problem presenting with vaginal discharge, soreness, anal pain, or bleeding. Behavioural changes such as encopresis or academic failure are unlikely to present at an A & E department.

There are important points to remember in the management of children with suspected sexual abuse.

1. Genital examination constitutes further abuse and should be limited to one experienced doctor. Every hospital to which children may be brought should have access to a doctor experienced in child sexual abuse.

2. Important evidence may be lost or distorted by inexperienced doctors. The role of the A & E senior house officer is to ensure the patient's general health and to contact more experienced colleagues.

Management of child presenting with acute perineal injury (straddle injury)

These children usually arrive with a history of having fallen astride a hard object. In most cases this history will be true, but in a few it is an attempt to conceal recent sexual abuse. There are two important questions to ask about children who are brought in with acute perineal trauma.

1. Is there a need for surgical intervention to control bleeding or repair damage?
2. Is the injury a result of sexual abuse?

The child's general well-being should be assessed first. Blood pressure and pulse should be noted and an assessment made of any blood lost. Other bruising or injury should be looked for. If there is blood loss, a brief visual inspection of the genital area is appropriate. This is to see if there is obvious severe trauma requiring emergency management. All children with any genital bleeding must be referred to the surgical department for consideration of examination under anaesthetic to exclude or treat vaginal or rectal tears. The examination will preferably be undertaken together with a forensic surgeon experienced in child sexual abuse. The child with perineal bruising only should be referred to the paediatric department for an opinion.

Management of child presented as having been raped

Occasionally a child, usually a girl, will be brought to the A & E department with a history of having ben raped. These patients must be examined that day by a forensic surgeon experienced in child sexual abuse. After an overall assessment to ensure the child's well-being, no attempt at genital examination should be performed until the forensic surgeon has arrived. No evidence, such as clothing, should be removed or disposed of, and the child should not be cleansed. The forensic surgeon will examine the patient and take appropriate specimens. He will arrange investigation for genital infection and post-coital contraception if appropriate.

In the meantime, however, the child should be comforted and reassured.

Presentation of chronic child sexual abuse

Chronic child sexual abuse is not a situation best dealt with by emergency referral out of hours. Children who have been brought to A & E because they have disclosed sexual abuse or in whom an adult suspects sexual abuse should be referred to the social services department. An arrangement will then be made for the child to be interviewed and examined by professionals expert in this difficult field.

The following symptoms usually have simple physical causes, but in a few children they will have arisen from repeated sexual abuse.

Presentation with local symptoms

1. Vulval soreness. The symptom is very common in pre-pubertal girls, and may be due to under- or over-hygiene or fungal infection. If the condition does not respond to simple measures (see p. 206) the child should be referred to paediatric out-patients.

2. Vaginal discharge. This may be caused by infection or occasionally by a foreign body. Swabs should be taken, including those for gonorrhoea and chlamydia. Antibiotics should not be given until the infection, if any, is identified. The child should be referred early to the paediatric out-patient department. The identification of a sexually transmitted disease in a child, although uncommon, is presumptive evidence of sexual abuse.

3. Anal bleeding and pain. This is usually caused by anal fissure related to constipation. Most will respond to laxatives, but referral back to the child's GP or to the paediatric out-patient department is necessary.

4. Perineal warts. These may be caused by self-inoculation from the fingers but may also be sexually transmitted. Children with perineal warts should be referred to the paediatric department.

Neglect (psychosocial deprivation)

In addition to failure to thrive (which should be assessed using standard percentile charts) neglected children may show certain well-recognized physical signs:

- small size as well as poor weight
- sparse dry hair

- protuberant abdomen
- cold red or blue extremities (acrocyanosis) even in a warm environment
- physically apathetic but wary ('frozen watchfulness')
- unresponsive to mother/carer.

Such children should be referred to the paediatric team.

Less common types of abuse

Children will sometimes present to the A & E department with unexplained coma, drowsiness, or apnoeic spells. Clearly, these children will be admitted under paediatric care. A few of them may have been intentionally poisoned or suffocated. It is wise to preserve samples of urine, vomit, and blood for further analysis from these children.

Munchausen syndrome by proxy is a condition in which factitious illness, for example spurious haematuria and induced rashes, is induced in a child by an adult. The condition usually takes some time to diagnose, and its recognition is often preceded by months of hospital admission and unnecessary investigation.

Further reading

1. Meadow, R. (ed.) (1989). *ABC of child abuse*. British Medical Journal, London.
2. MacCarthy, D. (1974). Effects of emotional disturbance and deprivation on somatic growth. In *Scientific foundations of paediatrics* (ed. J. Davies and J. Dobbing). Heinemann, London.

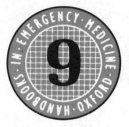

CHAPTER 9

Respiratory and ENT problems

Key points in respiratory disease

1 The severity of acute respiratory disease is best assessed by observation of the child's work of breathing and his state of alertness.

2 The child with respiratory disease who is drowsy or agitated is probably hypoxic. Pulse oximetry is a useful tool to assess hypoxia.

3 Respiratory disease is more likely to be severe in infants under the age of one year

4 Inspiratory stridor is always a serious symptom.

Presentation of respiratory disease

● Prevalence   Symptoms and signs

Prevalence

Respiratory disease is the most common cause of acute illness in childhood. Respiratory illness accounts for 50 per cent of consultations with GPs about children under five years of age and 30 per cent of consultations about 5–12 year olds.

Most infections (about 80 per cent) are limited to the upper respiratory tract (colds, pharyngitis, tonsillitis, otitis), but about 20 per cent affect the lower airway and respiratory tract (croup, epiglottitis, bronchitis, bronchiolitis, pneumonia) and are potentially more serious.

Asthma is the most common chronic disease of childhood and the most common single cause of admission of children to hospital.

Symptoms and signs of respiratory disease

Children with respiratory disease usually present with one or more of the following symptoms—cough, wheeze, stridor, breathlessness, or pyrexia. In addition, infants may present as generally unwell with poor feeding or occasionally with apnoeic spells. Older children with pneumonia may present with abdominal pain or chest pain on respiration. When taking the history it is important to be clear about what a parent is describing. For example, if a mother says 'His breathing is noisy', you need to ascertain whether she means wheeze, stridor, or the rattle of mucus in the airways.

The diagnosis of acute respiratory disease in childhood is largely clinical. It rests on history and examination, with a chest radiograph in some cases.

When assessing a child with a respiratory illness, three questions should be addressed.

1. What respiratory illness does the child have?
2. How severely affected is he by this illness?
3. What is the likely progression of the illness?

In assessing the symptoms and physical signs of acute respiratory disease the following should be noted.

1. *Nasal discharge*, which may be clear or mucopurulent with a cold.
2. *The characteristics of a cough*—is it barking, paroxysmal, or productive?
3. *Tachypnoea* indicates that increased ventilation is needed because of lung or airway disease (normal rate for infants

is 40–50 per minute). Tachypnoea may also be a sign of metabolic acidosis, severe infection, shock, diabetes, aspirin poisoning, or cardiovascular disease.

4. *Intercostal, subcostal, or sternal recession* shows increased work of breathing. This sign is more frequently seen in younger children who have a more plastic chest wall. Its presence in older children suggests moderate to severe lung disease. The degree of recession gives an indication of the severity of the respiratory difficulty.

5. The use of the sternomastoid muscle as an *accessory respiratory muscle* shows an increased work of breathing (in infants this may cause the head to bob up and down).

6. An inspiratory noise while breathing (*stridor*) is a sign of laryngeal or tracheal obstruction. In severely affected children stridor may occur also in expiration, but the inspiratory element is more prominent.

7. A *wheeze* indicates lower airways narrowing and is more prominent in expiration.

8. A *prolonged expiratory phase* indicates lower airways narrowing.

9. *Grunting* is caused by a child exhaling against a partially closed glottis in an attempt to generate a positive end expiratory pressure. It is a sign of severe respiratory distress and is usually seen only in infants.

10. *Flaring of the alae nasi* is seen particularly in infants with respiratory distress.

11. *Tachycardia* will be produced by hypoxia, anxiety, and fever.

12. *Pulsus paradoxus* is an exaggerated fall in pulse pressure during inspiration and is a sign of severe air trapping. It is detected on palpating the pulse volume.

13. Auscultatory findings; *rhonchi* (wheezes) indicate partial obstruction of medium airways and *crepitations* (crackles) are usually thought to indicate opening of partially obstructed bronchioles.

Alarming signs requiring urgent treatment:

• restlessness, agitation, drowsiness, or hypotonia in association with respiratory distress indicate hypoxia;
• central cyanosis is a late sign of very severe hypoxia.

Note: In infancy the main respiratory effort is diaphragmatic and so abdominal movement is more prominent than chest movement during breathing. Severe respiratory difficulty in a baby may produce a 'see-saw' pattern of breathing as the abdomen distends during inspiration and at the same time the chest retracts.

Causes of respiratory infections

The peak incidence of respiratory tract infection comes between two and four years of age. Children of this age may have up to ten respiratory illnesses a year. Parental smoking, overcrowded living conditions, and a history of prematurity significantly increase the frequency and severity of a child's respiratory infections.

Most respiratory infections are due to viruses, but it is often difficult to distinguish between viral and bacterial causes of infection either clinically or radiologically. Respiratory syncytial virus (RSV) is the most widely found respiratory virus but other important respiratory viruses include para-influenza viruses, influenza viruses, rhinoviruses, and adenoviruses. Important bacterial pathogens are haemolytic streptococci, which cause some cases of tonsillitis and pharyngitis, *Streptococcus pneumoniae*, which may cause otitis media or pneumonia, and *Mycoplasma pneumoniae*, which causes pneumonia usually in older children.

Upper respiratory infections

- **Coryzal illnesses (colds) Otitis media Otitis externa Sore throat**

Coryzal illnesses (colds)

Older children with colds rarely present to the A & E department as parents usually recognize these illnesses as self-limiting and benign. Young babies with colds may have difficulty with feeding because of their blocked noses, and medical advice may be sought. Mechanical clearing of the nose is usually best and can be done with a cotton bud or by tickling inside the baby's nose with a fine twist of cotton wool. A sneeze will rid the baby of mucus. Ephedrine vasoconstrictor nasal drops are not recommended as their effect is short and there may be worsening of the nasal mucosal swelling as the effect of the drug wears off. Frequent use of these nose drops can cause chemical rhinitis. The parents of babies with colds should be advised to feed their baby smaller amounts more frequently so that the infant has an overall adequate fluid intake. Children with systemic symptoms may need an antipyretic and analgesic, such as paracetamol, regularly for the first day or so.

Note: A runny nose is sometimes the first symptom of acute laryngotracheobronchitis, bronchiolitis, or pneumonia. In addition, viral upper respiratory tract infections are a common trigger of acute asthma. Parents of children who are discharged with a cold or sore throat should understand that they should seek further medical advice if their child develops new symptoms such as a barking cough, noisy breathing, or breathlessness. This is particularly important in the case of infants under one year old who are candidates for bronchiolitis and pneumonia. Children with a 'persistent cold' usually have allergic rhinitis and often have a person or family history of atopic disease. They should be referred back to their GP for treatment.

Otitis media

Infants and young children are prone to middle-ear infections. If improperly treated, these illnesses can cause partial deafness which may slow speech development in infants and cause poor concentration in the child at school.

Otitis media presents with a complaint of a painful ear in an older child. In a young child the presentation is less specific, and may be of vomiting, pyrexia, irritability, or pulling of the ear. The diagnosis is made by examination of the tympanic membranes. The normal drum is smooth, flat, and shiny. The inflamed drum is reddened (this may be just peripherally in the early stages), dull, and may be bulging or perforated. A yellow or white appearance is due to pus in the middle ear. The eardrum can look pink in a crying child but if uninfected it will remain shiny. Wax in the external auditory canal may obscure an inflamed eardrum.

Treatment of otitis media In addition to respiratory viruses, the organisms usually found in otitis media are *Streptococcus pneumoniae*, *Haemophilus influenzae*, and possibly *Branhamella catarrhalis*. Amoxycillin, co-trimoxazole, or a cephalosporin are generally effective. All cases of otitis media should be treated with systemic antibiotics so that bacterial infections are not left untreated.

Otitis externa

There is often profuse discharge from the ear in otitis externa, making it difficult to see the eardrum and therefore to distinguish between otitis externa and otitis media (pain which stops when the ear starts to discharge is usually caused by a perforated eardrum). Pulling at the pinna to straighten the external auditory canal during the examination sometimes produces pain in otitis externa but not in otitis media. In otitis externa, skin flora and *Pseudomonas aeruginosa* are the usual infecting organisms and treatment is with local antibiotic and steroid drops, such as Otosporin or Sofradex.

Sore throat

Sixty per cent of sore throats are caused by viral infections. The majority of the remainder are caused by Group A beta haemolytic streptococci. Streptococcal infection is uncommon in children under three years of age.

Infectious mononucleosis can affect children of all ages. The condition should be considered when a sore throat with exudate is accompanied by a measles-like rash and lymphadenopathy. An enlarged spleen may be palpable. The diagnosis can be confirmed by a Monospot test and the appearance of characteristic mononuclear cells on a blood film.

Herpangina is caused by Coxsackie viruses, and is characterized by fever and sore throat with vesicles or ulcers on the fauces.

Pharyngoconjunctival fever is caused by adenoviruses. The patient has fever, headache, conjunctivitis, and pharyngitis.

Scarlet fever caused by the erythrogenic beta haemolytic streptococcus will present with a rash accompanying a sore throat. In this case the rash is uniformly red and accompanied by a sore tongue with enlarged papillae. Occasionally pathognomonic striae may be seen on the flexor aspect of the elbows, and as the disease resolves there may be peeling of the palms.

Treatment of sore throats   There is no simple way of differentiating viral from bacterial causes of sore throat clinically. An exudate can be present in both viral and bacterial tonsillitis. A petachial rash on the palate can be seen with both streptococcal infection and glandular fever. A differential white cell count is unhelpful. If the child also has a runny nose, a viral infection is more likely. Antibiotics are usually given to children with marked tonsillar enlargement and those who are systemically unwell. if a decision is made on clinical grounds to give an antibiotic, oral penicillin is the drug of choice. For a patient who is sensitive to penicillin, erythromycin is the alternative choice.

Acute laryngotracheal disease

- Croup   Acute epiglottitis

The hallmark of disease of the larynx and trachea is an inspiratory stridor which may be accompanied by variable degrees of respiratory distress.

Croup

The term 'croup' is often used rather loosely to describe acute illnesses in which cough, inspiratory stridor, and respiratory distress occur. The different entities have different natural histories and require different management. Therefore they are described separately.

1. Acute laryngotracheobronchitis is by far the most common type of croup. It is caused by a virus, mainly para-influenza but also RSV, and occasionally measles or mumps. The disease usually begins as a coryza followed by the rather abrupt onset of stridor and barking cough, often commencing in the night. Most children with acute laryngotracheobronchitis are only mildly affected, and the most striking clinical feature in them is a frequent barking cough. A few children will have moderate to severe respiratory distress, and a small percentage of these will need intubation (see

p. 17). Most children will recover without treatment in two to five days.

2. Recurrent croup—some children, often with a personal or family history of atopy, have repeated episodes of croup without pyrexia or coryza. Hyper-reactivity of the upper airway may be the basis for their recurrent symptoms. In practice, it is difficult to distinguish an individual episode from the more common viral acute laryngotracheobronchitis.

3. Bacterial tracheitis—this is an unusual cause of croup but has a high mortality if untreated. The child will look toxic but has a croupy cough, unlike the child with epiglottitis. The usual infecting organisms are *Staphylococcus aureus* and *Haemophilus influenzae*. Intubation is usually required.

4. Tonsillitis—very rarely marked tonsillar enlargement, particularly with glandular fever, or abscess formation with a streptococal infection (quinsy) may cause an illness similar to mild epiglottitis. However, in these cases the obstruction is retropharyngeal rather than supraglottic. Intubation may be required.

5. Diphtheria—this is now a very uncommon cause of croup but should be considered in any non-immunized child.

6. Laryngeal foreign body—mechanical obstruction is less common than infection as a cause of acute stridor. However, the possibility of a foreign body should be considered in any case of stridor as its inhalation is often unwitnessed and therefore no inhalation history is given. For management see p. 185.

7. Angioneurotic oedema—laryngeal swelling occasionally occurs in acute anaphylactic reactions. For management see p. 40.

Acute epiglottitis

Acute epiglottitis is always a paediatric emergency. It needs immediate recognition and treatment, as the untreated disease carries a very high mortality. Acute epiglottitis is caused by *Haemophilus influenzae* type B and results in rapid swelling of the epiglottis and obstruction of the larynx. It requires urgent, but experienced, airway control. *Certain clinical features of epiglottitis can alert the A & E senior house officer to summon senior anaesthetic, ENT, and paediatric help immediately.*

- Very painful throat, unable to talk or drink, with drooling of saliva.
- Pale, ill-looking child with a fever.
- Quiet 'snoring' stridor.
- No barking cough (unlike acute laryngotracheobronchitis).
- Marked respiratory distress with tachypnoea, tachycardia, and sternal retraction.
- The patient often sits with his chin slightly elevated to optimize airway opening.

Assessment of the child with stridor Two main questions need to be addressed.

1. How severe is the upper airways obstruction and is it worsening?
2. Does the child have epiglottitis? (See above for clinical features.)

Assessment of severity Note: Never examine the throat of a patient with stridor as this procedure may precipitate respiratory arrest.

1. The degree of tachypnoea, sternal, and subcostal recession shows how much respiratory effort is needed to ventilate across the airway obstruction. *Caution:* A slowing respiration rate and reduction in recession with the onset of drowsiness show that the child is tiring and respiratory arrest is imminent.
2. Tachycardia and agitation are signs of increasing hypoxia. Central cyanosis indicates profound hypoxia.
3. The loudness of the stridor gives no indication of the severity of the obstruction.
4. The initial assessment of a child with stridor is entirely clinical. Investigations such as full blood count, throat swab, and lateral X-ray of the neck are unhelpful, and the procedures can precipitate complete obstruction by upsetting the child.

Management of acute airways obstruction If the child has marked respiratory distress, the aims of A & E management are as follows:

- improve oxygenation by giving a high concentration of oxygen by face mask;
- prevent the child becoming agitated, which will worsen hypoxia and possibly laryngeal oedema;
- involve senior experienced staff appropriately.

The parent's lap is a more reassuring place for the child than an A & E stretcher, and the parent is the best person to administer facial oxygen via a mask. A pulse oximeter will usefully monitor the patient's pulse rate and oxygen saturation if the child will tolerate the instrument on a digit.

Injections should not be given, and intravenous cannulae must not be inserted as they may precipitate acute obstruction by upsetting the child. Nebulized adrenalin (5 ml of 1:1000 adrenalin nebulized with oxygen) can be helpful in in obtaining transient improvement in children with severe obstruction while awaiting senior help. There is no objective evidence that water vapour is helpful in acute upper airways obstruction and it should not be used in the A & E department. There is some recent evidence for the use of inhaled budesonide in croup. In intensive care, parental steroids may be given to shorten the duration of intubation.

Intubation All children with epiglottitis, and about 2 per cent of hospitalized children with acute laryngotracheobronchitis, will require intubation. The decision to do this will be based on severely worsening respiratory distress or on the appearance of exhaustion, cyanosis, or confusion. Intubation of these children is very difficult and should not be undertaken by inexperienced doctors unless there has been a respiratory arrest.

Referral

1. Severely affected children (those with marked recession, exhaustion, confusion, or cyanosis)—*senior anaesthetic, paediatric, and ENT help should be obtained immediately* while ensuring good oxygenation, gentle handling, and administration of nebulized adrenalin.

2. Moderately affected children (those with stridor and recession at rest)—*paediatric referral should be made as soon as possible* so that the paediatrician may have an opportunity of assessing the child early.

3. Mildly affected children (barking cough, stridor on exertion only)—these should also be referred to the paediatrician.

No child with stridor should be discharged by junior A & E staff. Stridor is usually a symptom of sudden onset, and therefore the patient usually presents early in the evolution of the disease. The condition may worsen before it improves. The younger the child the more caution should be observed.

Lower respiratory infections

• **Bronchiolitis Pneumonia Bronchitis Whooping cough**

Bronchiolitis

Bronchiolitis is a viral infection of the small airways usually caused by RSV. It mainly affects infants under one year old and occurs in epidemics in the winter. The disease starts with a coryza and mild fever and progresses to wheeze, dry cough, and respiratory distress. The sicker infants will have respiratory rates over 60 per minute, marked recession, flaring alae nasi, and difficulty in feeding because of tachypnoea. They will be mildly hypoxic. A very few infants become exhausted, with slower respiration, severe hypoxia, and ventilatory failure. Apnoeic spells are a manifestation of the disease, particularly in young babies and those who have been born prematurely. These spells may be prolonged and frequent, and are sometimes an indication for ventilation.

In bronchiolitis, examination of the chest reveals hyperinflation which is also shown by an easily palpable liver. On auscultation there are widespread expiratory rhonchi and showers of fine inspiratory crepitations in the lungs.

Management and referral *Pale, tired, and tachypnoeic babies should be given oxygen immediately and referred to the paediatrician.* Many babies, despite mild tachypnoea, are cheerful and well. However, most babies with bronchiolitis should be admitted. This is because the condition takes several days to resolve and usually worsens before it improves, and babies may become exhausted before the condition is better. The exception to this is the baby who has had the illness for several days, has not had much difficulty in feeding, and is clearly recovering.

Pneumonia

Pneumonia can be a cause of death in very young or debilitated infants, or in children with underlying immuno-deficiency, respiratory, cardiac, or neuromuscular disease. However, most children with pneumonia have a mild disease and can be treated at home. The causative organisms in the child under five years of age are usually the respiratory viruses. *Streptococcus pneumoniae* is the most common bacterium identified and *Haemophilus influenzae* is an occasional pathogen. In children over five years old viral infection is rather less frequent, *Streptococcus pneumoniae* seems of greater importance, and *Mycoplasma pneumoniae* becomes more common. Pneumonia may present with some of the following symptoms:

- cough, initially dry then often productive
- wheeze—especially in children with viral infections
- pyrexia
- respiratory difficulty with tachypnoea and recession.

More rarely, the following symptoms may occur:

- abdominal pain—lower lobar pneumonia sometimes presents like this
- shoulder pain from diaphragmatic pleurisy
- pleuritic pain on inspiration

Points to note in the history   Enquiry should be made as to whether the child has an underlying chronic or congenital illness or was preterm. The history of the present illness and whether it is improving or worsening should be noted, together with what treatment has been received and specific enquiries about respiratory symptoms. Ask about the possibility of inhaled foreign body or food.

Points to note on examination
1. Is the child in respiratory distress, as shown by tachypnoea, recession, and the use of accessory muscles?
2. Is he pyrexial?

3. Does he look 'ill?'

4. What are the auscultatory findings?

Investigation It is difficult to distinguish between bacterial and viral pneumonia clinically or radiologically, and a differential white cell count is not helpful. Bacterial and viral infections may coexist in some cases. A chest X-ray should be performed if pneumonia is suspected clinically. A higher level of clinical suspicion for pneumonia should arise for children who have been preterm, have underlying cardio-respiratory disease, and in infants under the age of one year.

Referral Children in whom pneumonia is suspected or has been shown should be referred to the paediatrician. Not all will require admission.

Treatment Most children with a diagnosis of pneumonia are treated with antibiotics.

Penicillin or amoxycillin is usually prescribed unless the child has a typical history of *Mycoplasma pneumoniae* with headache and joint pains associated with the respiratory symptoms. In this case, or in a child failing to improve with penicillin, erythromycin should be used. A seven-day course of antibiotics is usually prescribed, and a repeat chest radiograph and out-patient review is arranged for a few weeks time.

Bronchitis

There is no clear clinical definition of bronchitis. The illness usually labelled 'bronchitis' is a cough, often with sputum, which accompanies a coryzal illness. This can be treated with penicillin or erythromycin, although many children improve without this treatment as the majority of pathogens are viral. Children with so-called 'recurrent bronchitis' often have asthma, and a trial of asthma medication under the supervision of their GP is warranted. There is no place for cough suppressants, linctuses, or expectorants in the treatment of 'bronchitis'.

Whooping cough

Despite the availability of pertussis immunization, whooping cough remains a common disease in children as immunization uptake is still not complete.

The disease usually starts uneventfully with a coryza and non-paroxysmal cough, but instead of resolving the cough worsens and becomes nocturnal, paroxysmal, and emetic. The characteristic whoop (an indrawing of breath at the end of an exhausting coughing paroxysm) is not always heard and is rarely noted in infants. During paroxysms, children become red in the face and may become cyanosed for short spells. Clear or white mucus is often expectorated. After a severe coughing spell conjunctival haemorrhages may appear and petechiae may be noted on the face. Children with whooping cough are not 'ill' between coughing and vomiting spells, but they may be tired because of disturbed sleep. The diagnosis is made by a history of persistence of the characteristic cough for several weeks, but may be supported in the early stages by a markedly raised lymphocyte count and confirmed by the isolation of *Bordetella pertussis* from a pernasal swab.

No treatment has been shown to be effective for established whooping cough. Erythromycin, given orally for 10 days in standard doses, is effective at clearing the naso-pharynx of organisms and therefore reducing infectivity. Erythromycin given to contacts who are still only in the coryzal phase may shorten the course of the illness but it has no clinical effect in the established case. It is worth giving the antibiotic to infant siblings of the index case. The GP should be asked to prescribe this.

Infants under six months of age who present to A & E with pertussis should be referred to the paediatric department for consideration of admission. These small babies may have apnoea and bradycardia with their coughing spells. The majority of deaths occur in this age group. In addition, children who have underlying chronic disease or who are severely socially disadvantaged are at risk from pertussis and should be referred to the paediatric department.

In general, however, otherwise healthy children over six months of age are as safe and less miserable when cared for at home and rarely need admission.

Asthma

- **Assessment of the asthmatic child presenting at the A & E department   Asthma: history   Asthma: examination   Investigations   Treatment   Referral**

Asthma is the most common chronic disorder of childhood. The prevalence of asthma seems to be increasing. Although new inhalation devices for treating asthma in children have become available, mortality has not decreased over the last 10 years and there has been a striking increase in the number of hospital admissions for asthma, particularly in children under five years of age.

Assessment of the asthmatic child presenting at the A & E department

The clinical picture of the child's asthmatic attack will be built up from a history, examination, and some simple investigations. However, *a distressed asthmatic child should receive face-mask oxygen and nebulized bronchodilators on arrival*, and not wait until all details have been assessed.

Asthma: history

1. How long has this episode lasted?
2. How bad has the child been? Has he been able to talk?
3. What medication has already been taken in this attack, by what route, and with what effect?
4. What asthma medication is the child regularly taking?
5. How frequent are the child's asthma symptoms usually?
6. Has the child had any previous severe attacks requiring steroid treatment, hospitalization, or intensive care?
7. Is there any identifiable trigger factor precipitating this episode?
8. Does the child have any other illnesses?

Asthma: examination

1. Increased work of breathing is a reliable indicator of severity. Signs include the use of accessory muscles and nasal flaring.

2. Decreased respiratory compliance is shown by recession. The younger the child the more readily this will occur, and it may be seen in several sites—subcostal, intercostal, sternal, and suprasternal.

3. The degree of wheeze is an unreliable sign in the assessment of asthma severity. Severely affected patients usually make little noise because their air flow is not high enough.

4. The restless agitated child is hypoxic. Cyanosis is a late sign of hypoxia.

5. Inability to speak, or sentences broken by pauses for breath, are signs of severe respiratory distress.

6. A raised pulse rate 40 or more points above base level indicates moderate to severe asthma, probably with hypoxia. A rate of over 150 indicates severe hypoxia or possibly beta-agonist excess.

7. The presence of pulsus paradoxus (exaggerated fall in pulse pressure during inspiration) is a sign of severe air trapping. However, the absence of pulsus paradoxus should not be taken as indicating mild disease.

8. Features of severe and life-threatening asthma are given in Boxes 9.1 and 9.2.

Box 9.1 **Features of severe asthma**

- Unable to talk in sentences
- Recession
- Peak flow below 50% of expected

Box 9.2 **Features of life-threatening asthma**

- Conscious level depressed
- Severe recession
- Marked use of accessory muscles
- Oxygen saturation less than 85% in air
- Peak flow less than 33% of expected
- Silent chest
- Cyanosis

Investigations

1. The peak flow rate is a very useful measurement in acute asthmatic attacks in patients old enough to use the equipment (usually over 5 or 6-years-old).

2. The non-invasive pulse oximeter is useful and can demonstrate minor degrees of desaturation undetectable clinically.

3. Estimations of arterial blood gases should be obtained in the most severely affected children, but the investigation must not delay treatment.

4. A chest radiograph is not usually helpful and may delay treatment. It should only be performed if there is poor response to treatment or there are auscultatory findings suggestive of localized respiratory pathology. A chest radiograph should be taken to look for pneumothorax if there is subcutaneous emphysema.

Treatment

Oxygen   Oxygen must be administered via a face mask to all hypoxic asthmatic patients. Asthmatic patients are often surprisingly hypoxic as ventilation–perfusion mismatch is added to airways obstruction.

β_2-**Agonists—salbutamol**   A nebulized broncholdilator, such as salbutamol (2.5 mg for children under seven and 5 mg for children over seven), should be given in 5 ml of normal saline. The flow rate for air or oxygen should be 8 litres/min and the patient should be instructed to breathe through his mouth. A poor or short-lived response is a bad sign; a further dose can be given immediately but the paediatrician should be called urgently. Continuous nebulized bronchodilator can be given in severe cases.

Aminophylline   If the child fails to improve with nebulized salbutamol, intranveous aminophylline (5 mg/kg) can be given by the doctor over 20 minutes while monitoring the pulse rate. This should be followed by an infusion of aminophylline at 1 mg/kg/h. Aminophylline can cause ventricular arrhythmias if given quickly and may also cause nausea and vomiting. If the child has had a short-acting theophylline preparation in the previous six hours or a long-acting one in the previous 18 hours, the loading dose should be omitted and the infusion dose only used. If the child feels nauseous, the infusion should be slowed down, and it should be stopped if pulse irregularities occur. Patients on intravenous aminophylline must continue to have two-hourly nebulized salbutamol or terbutaline, and oxygen continuously.

Steroids   Steroids speed up recovery from acute asthma. A dose of 2 mg/kg oral prednisone should be given. Intravenous hydrocortisone is only necessary if the patient is vomiting or unable to take the oral drug. Further doses may be given on subsequent days.

Antibiotics   Antibiotics are rarely required in acute asthmatic episodes.

Referral

Patients in severe respiratory distress and those responding poorly, or not at all, to nebulized salbutamol and oxygen should be referred urgently to the paediatricians.

   No child must be allowed home immediately after receiving nebulized salbutamol or terbutaline. Although marked clinical improvement may occur following this treatment, it may be short-lived and the patient be just as bad again, or worse, in a few hours. Therefore it follows that, unless the A & E department or paediatric ward has appropriate child-oriented facilities for observation for a few hours, children who have had nebulized bronchodilators will require admission. If there are facilities for observation, the child can be reassessed in approximately four hours. If the clinical response is maintained, the child is not wheezy, and the peak flow has not fallen again, he may be allowed home with a suitable β-agonist for inhalation, using a large volume spacer device or a turbohaler, every four to six hours over the next 48–72 hours. The parents should be instructed to bring the child back if he worsens, and review should be arranged for the next day. Children who are on inhaled steroids should receive a three-day course of oral steroids in a dose of 2 mg/kg daily ('tailing off' of this course is not necessary). Other candidates for a short course of oral steroids are children whose asthma attack is not responding to treatment despite 24 hours of regular inhaled bronchodilator therapy every four to six hours at home.

It is important that the parent of a discharged asthmatic child understands that an apparent response to inhaled β-agonists does not mean the end of the asthma attack. Although the child may be apparently improved, he will continue with significant small airways obstruction for several days. Therefore treatment with inhaled β-agonists, and in many cases oral steroids, must be continued over this time on a regular basis and the parents told to bring the child back if he deteriorates. If the patient is discharged from the A & E department, his GP or paediatrician should be informed as an acute attack may be a failure of prophylaxis and signals the need to reconsider the patient's regular asthma treatment.

Patients who have been observed over four hours and who are again wheezy or whose peak flow has fallen will require admission.

Chronic cough

   • **Causes of chronic cough   Examination   Referral**

Occasionally a child with a chronic cough will attend an A & E department, particularly if the symptoms have just worsened acutely. A careful history and examination should indicate those who require further investigation and referral.

Causes of chronic cough

1. The most common cause is asthma, which in some mildly affected children will be manifested only as a cough. Supporting features for this diagnosis are that the cough is dry, worsens at night and on exercise, and may be associated with episodes of wheeze. There may be a history of atopy in the family, or eczema, urticaria, or allergic rhinitis in the child.

2. Whooping cough is characterized by a paroxysmal nocturnal emetic cough, sometimes accompanied by an inspiratory whoop (see p. 177).

3. Some children with apparent chronic cough will have frequent lower respiratory tract infections, perhaps associated with parental smoking, overcrowding in the home, or preterm delivery.

4. Some children develop a habit cough after a respiratory illness. The habit cough is notable for its honking quality, absence in sleep, absence of sputum, and accentuation when the child is anxious.

5. An inhaled foreign body is a less common cause of a usually productive cough (see p. 185).

   Rarer causes of chronic cough include the following.

6. Cystic fibrosis—this occurs in one in 2000 children, and is associated with poor weight gain and offensive stools.

7. Recurrent aspiration syndrome—causes repeated respiratory symptoms in infancy.

8. Immunodeficiency syndromes—recurrent serious infections should prompt a search for immune deficiency syndromes.

9. Tuberculosis—this infection produces wheezing and weight loss in childhood. However, some cases are discovered when a chest radiograph is ordered for a chronic cough or unrelated cause. The condition should be particularly remembered in children who live in immigrant communities.

Examination

The signs of chronic respiratory disease are as follows:

- poor growth.
- abnormally shaped chest with a Harrison's sulcus or a barrel shape.
- clubbing of the fingers.

All children with chronic cough should have a chest radiograph. A foreign body, tuberculosis, or radiological changes of chronic chest disease will be discovered in some. In asthma the chest radiograph will probably be normal. This investigation is not urgent and need not be done out of hours.

Referral

Referral to paediatric out-patients should be made for children with any physical signs of chest disease or abnormalities on their chest radiograph. Other children should be referred back to their GP who should be sent a copy of the X-ray report.

Chest pain

Unlike adults, the complaint of chest pain in children and adolescents rarely points to cardiac disease.

Following trauma, bruising or rib or sternal fractures are causes of chest pain. In a child with respiratory distress or a history of respiratory illness, such as asthma or cystic fibrosis, a pneumothorax is a possibility. Worsening of pain on inspiration or a pleural rub or dullness indicates pleurisy or an effusion. An oesophageal or bronchial foreign body can give rise to chest pain.

Congenital aortic stenosis occasionally gives rise to chest pain. The disease can be diagnosed by the finding of a left ventricular impulse, a murmur in the aortic area at the right first intercostal space transmitted into the neck, and a thrill in the suprasternal notch. In addition to history and examination, a chest radiograph should be useful in diagnosing any of these causes of chest pain.

Otherwise well patients with chest pain but no physical signs or chest radiograph abnormalities usually have viral myositis, oesophagitis, or psychosomatic chest pain. They should be referred back to their GP. If clinically indicated, an antacid can be prescribed for a child who has chest pain from oesophagitis.

Foreign bodies

- **Laryngeal foreign body**   **Intrabronchial foreign body**

Laryngeal foreign body

Obstruction of the larynx is one of the most common causes of accidental death in children under one year old. Children with a partially obstructing foreign body in the larynx present with stridor, a distressing cough, and variable degrees of respiratory distress. A history of choking on food or a toy is usual, but not inevitable, and the possibility of a laryngeal foreign body should be remembered in any case of stridor.

Management Management is described on p. 30. A swallowed foreign body (for general management see p. 148) may lodge in the upper oesophagus and produce dysphagia, drooling, and difficulty in speaking. Urgent surgical or ENT help should be obtained and the foreign body removed by oesophagoscopy.

Intrabronchial foreign body

An intrabronchial foreign body is more common than a laryngeal one and is very unlikely to be initially fatal. There is considerable delay in diagnosis in a third of cases. Eighty per cent of patients with a bronchial foreign body are less than four years old; peanuts comprise half of the inhaled objects.

Prompt presentation Children who present acutely following a choking episode usually have a sudden onset of wheeze and cough. There may be diminished breath sounds over the affected area of the lung.

Delayed presentation If choking was not noticed or was dismissed as unimportant, the patient may present days or weeks later with a cough, wheeze, and fever, unresolved pneumonia, or recurrent cough with haemoptysis. Delay in diagnosis at this stage is usually due to the doctor's not being aware that respiratory symptoms could be due to the inhalation of a foreign body.

Radiological investigation Most foreign bodies in the lung are not radio-opaque. However, the resulting collapse, hyperinflation, or consolidation is usually seen on a chest radiograph. The actual radiographic changes will depend on whether the obstruction is complete or partial and whether there has been additional infection. Films taken in both full expiration and full inspiration are necessary in the assessment of the presence of a foreign body. In a young child, if these films cannot be obtained easily, the chest and diaphragm should be screened.

Management Most bronchial foreign bodies can be removed at bronchoscopy. However, many children will have long-term pulmonary symptoms, particularly after delayed removal.

Further reading

1. Phelan, P. D., Landau, L. J., and Olinsky, A. (1990). *Respiratory illness in children* (3rd edn). Blackwell Scientific, Oxford.

CHAPTER 10

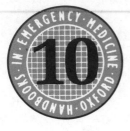

Gastrointestinal and genitourinary problems

Key points in gastrointestinal and genitourinary problems

1 Oral rehydration therapy is the mainstay of treatment in gastroenteritis.

2 Vomiting is a non-specific symptom of many illnesses, some of which are serious. A child should not be discharged with undiagnosed vomiting.

3 The concern in acute abdominal pain in childhood is whether appendicitis, or less frequently intussusception, is present.

4 There should be a high index of suspicion for urinary tract infections in infants and young children. All children with urinary tract infection or haematuria must be followed up.

Gastrointestinal and genitourinary problems

Diarrhoea, vomiting, and abdominal pain are the most common gastrointestinal symptoms with which children present to A & E departments.

Gastroenteritis and chronic diarrhoea

• **Gastroenteritis   Chronic diarrhoea**

Gastroenteritis

Gastroenteritis is a major cause of death in children worldwide, but in the UK it is usually a relatively mild condition, and has become milder over the last 10 years. The decrease in severity is attributed to earlier use of oral rehydration therapy (ORT) and fewer cases of hypernatraemic dehydration resulting from a decrease in the solute content of formula milks.

Clinical presentation   Patients will present with diarrhoea, vomiting, or both. There may be abdominal pain, pyrexia, or blood in the stools. The following points should be clarified in the history:

• duration of symptoms
• number, volume, and description of stools and vomits
• number, volume, and type of feeds taken
• parent's assessment of child's well-being
• medication already received
• history of underlying disease
• affected contacts.

Examination   A full clinical examination is essential:

• to assess the degree of dehydration;
• to exclude other causes of diarrhoea or vomiting, e.g. acute abdomen, otitis media, meningitis, constipation with overflow.

The patient's weight must be recorded so that a baseline is available if he should return for follow-up.

Symptoms and signs of dehydration

1. Thirst—*Note*: a very ill baby may be too lethargic to suck.
2. Decreased urinary output—less than four wet nappies in the previous 24 hours suggests dehydration.
3. Dry mouth—a useful sign if the child is not a mouth breather.
4. Decreased skin turgor—this usually reliable sign may underestimate dehydration if hypernatraemia or obesity is present, or overestimate it in patients with hyponatraemia or malnutrition. Several sites, for example abdomen and inner arm, should be tested by pinching up the skin—any delay in return of the tested skin to normal indicates dehydration.
5. Sunken anterior fontanelle—this is a useful sign in infants, but some infants with a large anterior fontanelle always show some depression. Depression will be underestimated if the baby is crying or lying down.
6. Sunken eyes and decreased eyeball turgor—the latter is not an easy sign to elicit.
7. Tachypnoea—the metabolic acidosis of dehydration causes deep and rapid respiration.
8. Tachycardia—reduced circulatory volume will cause a rapid poor-volume pulse, but this sign is also present in ill children in general and is not specific for dehydration.
9. Child's demeanour—dehydrated children may be restless, lethargic, or irritable, but these are general signs of ill health.

For assessment of degree of dehydration see Table 10.1.

Table 10.1 • Assessment of dehydration

	Mild (<5%)	Moderate (5%–10%)	Severe (<10%)
Dry mouth	-	+	+
Reduced skin turgor	-	±	+
Sunken fontanelle	-	+	+
Sunken eyes	-	+	+
Tachypnoea	-	±	+
Tachycardia	-	±	+
Drowsiness	-	±	+

Stool specimens should be sent for bacteriology, parasites, and viral culture. Rapid tests are available for the diagnosis of rotavirus infection.

Indications for referral to paediatric care

1. Patients (usually infants) who are severely (more than 10 per cent) dehydrated with circulatory collapse. These infants are pale, floppy, and tachypnoeic, and have a rapid weak pulse. They should have an immediate intravenous infusion of 20 ml/kg of 5 per cent human albumin, or 0.9 per cent saline given over five minutes. The infusion should be repeated if there is little or no clinical improvement. Blood should be taken for electrolytes, a film (looking for evidence of disseminated intravascular coagulation or haemolysed red cells), culture, acid–base status, urea, haemoglobin, and white cell count. *Meanwhile urgent paediatric assistance should be sought.*

2. Patients who have clinical signs of moderate dehydration (5 per cent plus). These patients will probably be managed with ORT but need hospital observation.

3. Infants under three months of age. Gastroenteritis is less common in very young infants. They are at greater risk of dehydration, and systemic illness and other causes for their symptoms are more difficult to exclude.

4. Children for whom clinical exclusion of other causes of their symptoms is not certain. Particular traps to look for include the infant with pyloric stenosis who may have small loose 'starvation' stools as well as vomiting; superficially he may appear to have gastroenteritis. Also consider intussusception; the classical 'redcurrant jelly' stool is a late symptom.

5. Children with profuse vomiting and/or diarrhoea who might become more poorly.

6. Children whose parents are in your, or the GP's, view very anxious or unable to manage at home.

7. Children with a high fever.

8. Children with underlying chronic disease, for example sickle cell disease or immune deficiency.

Patients who do not require admission The majority of patients will be older infants and toddlers with no clinical evidence of dehydration and who are not 'ill'. The mainstays of treatment for these children are as follows:

- ORT
- early re-introduction of normal feeds and diet.

For a period of not more than 24 hours normal feeds and diet are replaced by a water-based solution of electrolytes and glucose. The exception is for babies who are being breast-fed. Breast-feeding should continue and ORT should be offered in addition after the breast feed. Intestinal absorption of sodium and water occurs by active transport utilizing glucose. Replacement of fluid and electrolytes lost through diarrhoea can be achieved by giving a solution of sodium, potassium, and glucose with bicarbonate or citrate to counter acidosis. It seems clear from a number of studies that a range of solute concentrations can be tolerated by children with gastroenteritis. The World Health Organization formulation contains 90 mmol sodium/litre, but this is probably more appropriate to clinically dehydrated children. Commercially available preparations such as Dextrolyte, Dioralyte, Gluco-Lyte, and Electrosol (all 35 mmol sodium/litre), and Electrolade and Rehidrat (50 mmol sodium/litre), are all satisfactory for out-patient use. Parents should be advised to give their child at least his normal daily fluid requirements as ORT (see Table 10.2). Extra ORT should be offered if he appears thirsty and following the passage of a watery stool. If the child is vomiting, small frequent feeds should be given. If vomiting continues despite this, admission will be necessary. It is important that the parent understands that ORT is not a medicine to 'cure' the diarrhoea (although a reduction in stool number is usual), but is to prevent dehydration and electrolyte imbalance. Normal baby milk feeds and then diet, if appropriate, are re-introduced after 24 hours (or earlier if the diarrhoea has settled or the child appears hungry). The re-introduction of feeds may cause an increase in the number or volume of stools, but further starvation is contra-indicated. It is preferable that the child's bowel absorbs some nutrients than none at all. Further ORT or watery drinks should be offered in addition to feeds and diet if diarrhoea continues. Highly sugary, carbonated, or·very cold drinks should be avoided, as these will affect gut motility and absorption.

Table 10.2 • Daily oral fluid requirements for well children

Age (yr)	0–1	1–3	4–6	7–14
Volume (ml/kg)	150	100	90	70

Follow-up Children should be reviewed at 24 hours. This should usually be arranged with the child's GP. Parents should be asked to return with their child before this appointment if:

• he seems more ill, especially if drowsy or pyrexial
• vomiting does not stop
• diarrhoea worsens.

At the review appointment the child should be reweighed and reassessed. Any anxieties at this stage should lead to a paediatric referral.

Rotavirus causes more than 50 per cent of cases of childhood gastroenteritis in the UK. Respiratory symptoms are often associated with viral or *Cryptosporidium* gastroenteritis. In recent arrivals to this country, illnesses endemic abroad such as cholera and amoebiasis must be considered. Shigella and campylobacter infections may cause bloody diarrhoea, and shigella infection may also provoke convulsions. Remember that salmonella and shigella infections are notifiable diseases.

Antibiotics and antidiarrhoeals There is no place for antibiotics in the home management of gastroenteritis. In the vast majority of cases gastroenteritis is a self-limiting disease in which antibiotics appear to prolong the illness. Anti-diarrhoeals (for example kaolin, Lomotil) of all types are always contraindicated as they mask symptoms, prolong disease, and cause side-effects in children.

Complications of gastroenteritis Diarrhoea persisting beyond two weeks indicates reinfection, prolonged infection (for example *Escherichia coli*, *Cryptosporidium*), secondary lactose intolerance, or cows' milk protein intolerance. Fresh stools should be sent for culture, pH, and sugar chromatography, and the child should be referred to the paediatric department.

Chronic diarrhoea

Some children present to A & E departments with long-standing diarrhoea. These children should be referred to the paediatric out-patient clinic.

If the child is symptom free apart from the diarrhoea, has no abnormality on physical examination, and is thriving, he may have 'toddler's diarrhoea' which is a disorder of bowel motility. The appearance of undigested vegetables in the stools is a feature of this condition. A non-urgent paediatric out-patient referral is appropriate. However, if he has additional symptoms or abnormal physical signs, or is failing to put on weight, urgent paediatric out-patient referral or admission would be appropriate. Conditions presenting like this with chronic diarrhoea are constipation with overflow, cystic fibrosis, coeliac disease, or sugar intolerances. In the older child, diarrhoea with blood or mucus in the stool suggests inflammatory bowel disease.

Acute abdominal pain

- **Common causes of acute abdominal pain in childhood**
  Appendicitis   Constipation   Rectal bleeding

Common causes of acute abdominal pain in childhood

- Acute non-specific abdominal pain (ANSAP). This is a diagnosis of exclusion but is still the most common diagnosis in children admitted to hospital with abdominal pain. The term really means that we cannot find a cause for the pain, and it ceases spontaneously.
- Acute appendicitis (see below)
- Constipation (see p. 197)
- Gastroenteritis (see p. 189)
- Intussusception (see p. 201)
- Urinary tract infection (see p. 202)
- Pneumonia (see p. 176)
- Diabetes (see p. 40)
- Henoch–Schonlein purpura (see p. 233)
- Sickle cell disease (see p. 238)

Appendicitis

The most usual concern in a child with acute abdominal pain is 'is this acute appendicitis or not?'

The suspicion that abdominal pain is due to appendicitis is based on a good history and examination. Investigations do not clarify an uncertain picture.

History—points to note

1. Previous similar bouts of pain make this one less likely to be appendicitis.

2. Appendicitis pain usually begins at low intensity either initially in the right lower quadrant or moving there from centrally. It becomes gradually more intense but is rarely agonizing. It is usually constant and less often colicky. It may improve a little with rest.

3. The child with appendicitis is usually not hungry but will drink.

4. A few vomits are usual but profuse vomiting is uncommon in uncomplicated appendicitis.

5. Although a history of constipation or diarrhoea may suggest an alternative cause for the abdominal pain, both bowel symptoms may coexist with appendicitis.

6. The duration of symptoms in appendicitis before the patient is seen may be from a few hours to several days depending on the state the disease has reached, and any modifying treatment, such as antibiotics or analgesics, that may have altered the natural history of the condition.

7. Remember to ask for the presence of symptoms that might indicate a different diagnosis, for example polyuria (diabetes) or a cough (pneumonia).

The physical examination Before embarking on the physical examination the patient should be made comfortable and reassured by a parent close at hand. Analgesics should not be given as they will mask clinical signs.

1. Start by assessing the patient in general—uncomplicated appendicitis produces a moderately ill child. A desperately ill child may have widespread peritonitis or a completely different diagnosis.

2. A normal temperature and pulse rate may be present in appendicitis and both will be raised in an acute infectious disease, so these measurements do not help in the differential diagnosis. However, they should be recorded as

changes may be useful. A rapid respiration rate is a useful sign as this suggests pneumonia or diabetes as a cause of the abdominal pain and should lead to a chest X-ray and blood sugar estimation.

3. Examination of the abdomen should start with inspection. The child should be asked to point to the area of pain—a vague indication of all over the abdomen is a pointer away from appendicitis.

4. Palpation should start well away from the area that the child says is painful. You are assessing tenderness and guarding. An area of tenderness and guarding at McBurney's point (two-thirds of the way from the umbilicus to the anterior superior iliac spine) is the classical sign of uncomplicated appendicitis. More widespread tenderness suggests peritonitis. Generalized guarding in a well child is more often a sign of anxiety than of peritonitis.

5. Halitosis is often absent in the younger child with appendicitis.

6. A rectal examination is not necessary if you have clearly decided to refer the child to the surgeon. He will want to repeat what is an unpleasant procedure for the child. However, in any case of doubt, a rectal examination should be performed to identify pelvic tenderness caused by a retrocaecal appendix or pelvic peritonitis.

7. Pain apparently arising in the right hip may be caused by a retrocaecal appendicitis causing psoas muscle spasm.

8. In doubtful cases it is helpful to ask the child to sit up, get off the examination couch, and jump up and down on the floor. A child who can quickly and happily perform these activities is unlikely to have serous abdominal pathology.

9. If your department has the facility, observation for three to four hours and then re-examination may be useful in doubtful cases.

Investigations Full blood count, abdominal X-ray, and urinalysis are not useful in distinguishing appendicitis from other causes of acute abdominal pain and, except for urinalysis, they should not be done routinely.

Referral At this stage children in whom you have made a firm diagnosis of appendicitis and children in whom doubt remains should be referred to the surgical team. Children with abdominal pain who are allowed home should be given a review appointment in 24 hours, but should be asked to return earlier if the pain worsens or new symptoms develop. Most cases of non-specific abdominal pain will settle in 24 hours.

Pitfalls in the diagnosis of acute appendicitis

1. The patient has been given antibiotics for a supposed infection. This may mask clinical signs—have a higher degree of suspicion in these patients.

2. The patient is receiving analgesics. Again, a higher degree of suspicion is needed.

3. Appendicitis in the toddler is unusual but usually presents late with complications because the child cannot complain of abdominal pain as clearly as the older child.

4. It is easy to underestimate the pain experienced by a stoical child and overestimate that experienced by an upset child. You need to spend a little time forming an impression of the child's response to pain.

5. There is sometimes a 'window' of absent clinical signs when an appendix has just burst and before peritonitis has set in.

Constipation

Constipation is a common condition in childhood and presents acutely in A & E departments as:

- acute abdominal pain.
- anal bleeding.

A history of infrequent evacuation of small hard stools may be obtained, but the diagnosis is made on palpating a loaded descending colon and finding the rectum full of hard faeces. Particularly in babies and young children an anal tear may initiate fear of evacuation and hence constipation occurs. Fresh blood on the stool is usually caused by an anal fissure. Children very rarely have haemorrhoids. An abdominal X-ray will show the extent of the loaded colon but is not necessary for the diagnosis of constipation. It is worth remembering that constipation is so common that it may coexist with other illnesses such as appendicitis. Hirschsprung's disease is uncommon, but should be considered in constipated children with a history of late passage of meconium when newborn, poor growth, or constipation unresponsive to treatment.

Treatment   If the child is in acute discomfort a micro-enema or a phosphate enema may be necessary to relieve him if he will tolerate the procedure. A few children with unresponsive constipation will need hospital admission, although where there is a paediatric District Nurse service home supervision is as effective. In most cases an oral stool softener such as lactulose is sufficient. Where lactulose has not been effective a laxative such as Senokot should be given. Patients with anal fissure will only need an oral stool softener. Advice on the usefulness of a high fibre diet should be given. The majority of patients should be followed up by their GP, but more severe cases should be referred to the paediatric out-patient department. Treatment for constipation is usually needed for at least several months to allow the stretched rectum to resume its normal size and elasticity.

Rectal bleeding

Although rectal bleeding is most commonly associated with constipation in childhood, other causes need to be considered and paediatric referral made.

1. Vitamin K deficiency in the newborn.
2. Shigella gastroenteritis—accompanied by diarrhoea.
3. Inflammatory bowel disease—usually in an older child. The history is of chronic diarrhoea with blood and/or mucus. There may be weight loss. Urgent paediatric out-patient referral is needed.
4. Intussusception—in the under 2-year-old rectal bleeding with abdominal pain is a potential surgical emergency (see p. 201).
5. Rarely, rectal bleeding may be the presenting feature of a clotting disorder. Ask for family history and look for abnormal bruising.
6. Again, rarely, more profuse rectal bleeding may originate from an intestinal polyp or Meckel's diverticulum.
7. Very occasionally rectal bleeding may be the initial presentation of sexual abuse (see p. 161).

Vomiting

Gastro-oesophageal reflux   Plyloric stenosis
Intussusception

Vomiting should be differentiated from possetting which is the regurgitation of mouthfuls of curdled milk in a young infant. Vomiting associated with winding of a baby suggests excessive swallowed air. A larger hole in the feeding bottle's teat will reduce the amount of air swallowed.

Vomiting is often a non-specific sign of illness in childhood. It may be a presenting symptom of the following:

- gastroenteritis (see p. 188)
- gastro-oesophageal reflux (see below)
- otitis media and tonsillitis (see p. 169–171)
- urinary tract infection (see p. 202)
- associated with a cough, for example whooping cough (see p. 177).

However, some causes of vomiting, although less common, are serious and should be actively considered:

- appendicitis (see p. 194)
- pyloric stenosis (see p. 200)
- intussusception (see p. 201)
- bowel obstruction, for example volvulus, adhesions from previous surgery, strangulated hernia (see p. 243)
- meningitis (see p. 216, 220)
- raised intracranial pressure from any cause
- Reye's syndrome (see p. 36).

No child should be allowed home with undiagnosed vomiting. Bile-stained vomiting should always lead to admission.

Gastro-oesophageal reflux

Gastro-oesophageal reflux is very common in infants. However, some infants vomit many times daily and treatment may be necessary until the condition spontaneously resolves with increasing maturity and the use of solid food. Most infants improve in the second six months of life.

Complications in more severe cases include recurrent

pulmonary aspiration, apnoeic spells, anaemia from gastro-intestinal blood loss, failure to thrive, and oesophageal stricture.

Occasionally gastrointestinal malrotation may mimic reflux—a short or intermittent history of vomiting should raise suspicion of this.

History There is often a long history of frequent vomiting, usually after feeds and on handling the baby. Babies with reflux vomit less when asleep than awake and most gain weight normally.

Examination The diagnosis of gastro-oesophageal reflux in A & E is from the history. In an uncomplicated case there are no abnormal physical signs.

Management An explanation of the cause of symptoms should be given to parents. A feed thickener (Carobel or Nestargel) should be prescribed.

Referral The baby's own GP should be informed and should continue management. In more severe cases refer to the paediatric out-patient department. Babies who are failing to gain weight require immediate paediatric referral.

Pyloric stenosis

Pyloric stenosis is more common in boys than in girls. There is a family history of the complaint in about 10 per cent of patients.

History Pyloric stenosis characteristically presents with a short history of forceful vomiting in a baby of two to eight weeks of age. The vomit may contain altered blood subsequent to gastritis. The baby may have had no stool for a day or so, or may be passing small loose 'starvation' stools.

Examination Depending on the length of history, the baby may be dehydrated or show evidence of recent weight loss. The upper abdomen may be distended and visible gastric peristalsis may be seen with patient observation. The diagnosis is made by the palpation of an evanescent olive-sized mass at the pylorus. This is most easily palpable while the baby is taking a milk feed. A hypochloraemic hypokalaemic metabolic alkalosis may be present. Pyloric stenosis should be considered in any vomiting baby less than three months old.

Referral The baby should be referred to the paediatric team for confirmation of the diagnosis and biochemical correction before surgery.

Intussusception

This condition is more common in children under two years of age. It presents as an acute onset of colicky abdominal pain, in some cases with vomiting. In late cases, findings are bloody stools and a palpable abdominal mass. Intussusception should be considered in any young child with acute abdominal pain, often seen as episodes of screaming with or without pallor. An abdominal X-ray may be helpful in showing fluid levels indicating obstruction, but a normal X-ray does not exclude the condition. Referral to the surgical team is indicated if the condition is suspected. The diagnosis is confirmed on barium enema, and the enema may be used to reduce the intussusception.

Recurrent abdominal pain

Children with recurrent abdominal pain may present to the A & E department with an acute episode of pain. It may be that the pain is particularly bad and the parents are concerned that this time there may be something seriously wrong. This may be the case and the patient should be assessed as for acute abdominal pain (see p. 194).

Recurrent abdominal pain is a common symptom in childhood, and in an otherwise well and thriving child with no other symptoms or signs than occasional vomits or a headache it is unusual for there to be any demonstrable physical pathology. The symptom may be stress-related, and there may be a family history of similar illness or of migraine.

Management Once acute abdominal pathology is excluded, a mid-stream clean voided urine sample should be taken and the parents and child reassured that no acute illness has been found. The child may be discharged from A & E. The GP should be informed and the parents advised to consult further with their child's GP.

Threadworms

Although not an emergency, children with threadworms may present at the A & E department in the night when parents observe the alarming sight of worms emerging from their child's anus. Threadworms are an innocuous infestation which cause perineal itching, particularly at night, and the diagnosis is made by observing the small thread-like white worms on perianal skin or in the stool. Piperazine is the standard treatment—one sachet stirred into a drink for children over five years of age and half this dose for younger children. The treatment may be repeated after 14 days. It is usual to treat siblings also, and this should be done by the family's GP.

Urinary tract infections

• Background   When to suspect a urinary tract infection

Background

An infection may be the first evidence of a treatable urinary tract abnormality. It is thought that renal damage in sufferers from chronic renal failure associated with reflux nephropathy is initiated with the first urine infection in early childhood. Therefore it is important that those caring for young children should recognize, treat, and investigate urinary tract infections (UTIs) appropriately. In early childhood, UTIs do not present as dysuria and frequency but as pyrexia, vomiting, or malaise. Therefore, examination of the urine is part of the examination of every child except those in whom a clear alternative diagnosis has been established.

When to suspect a urinary tract infection

Urine should be taken for culture in the following circumstances.

• In children who complain of dysuria, frequency, or suprapubic pain.
• In any febrile child in whom the cause of pyrexia is not found on examination.

- In any child with poor weight gain, vomiting, poor feeding, lethargy, or irritability (as part of full investigations).
- In children with haematuria.
- In febrile children with pain and tenderness in the renal area.
- In a sick neonate as part of a bacteriological work-up.
- In children with abdominal pain.
- In children whose parents have observed abnormalities of colour or smell in their urine.
- In children with enuresis.

The urine specimen To be correctly interpreted the urine specimen must be properly collected and examined within an hour by the laboratory. Specimens taken at night may be refrigerated or taken into a specimen pot containing the preservative boric acid.

Methods of urine collection are as follows.

1. Mid-stream clean voided urine (MSU)—this is the method of choice for collection from the continent child. Collecting the middle of the stream allows the urethral organisms to be flushed out before the specimen is taken. The perineum should be cleansed first with sterile water.

2. Bag specimens—this method is suitable only for the exclusion of UTI. A positive bag specimen should lead to a clean catch or suprapubic aspirate. The perineum must be cleansed before the bag is affixed and the patient must be kept upright; the bag must be removed as soon as urine has been passed.

3. Clean catch urine in infants—this requires patience on the part of nursing staff or parents. An adult must sit with the semi-naked baby until urine is passed, catching the middle of the stream in a sterile container. It is worth remembering that babies micturate at mealtimes, when handled, and usually about every two hours.

4. Suprapubic aspiration—this is needed in the sick neonate or young infant.

5. Catheter sample—this is sometimes necessary in handicapped older children who cannot produce a clean midstream specimen.

The diagnosis of a UTI is made when a culture shows more than 10^5 pure growth of a urinary pathogen in a correctly collected and handled urine specimen. A single catheter or suprapubic specimen is adequate to diagnose a UTI, but other methods of collection require at least two samples.

The presence of large numbers of pus cells or red cells in the urine may be suggestive of a UTI, but is not diagnostic and their absence certainly does not exclude UTI. The presence or absence of protein is unhelpful. Bacteria visible on microscopy are strongly suggestive of UTI.

Treatment When UTI has been diagnosed a seven-day course of an antibiotic to which the organism is sensitive should be given. If the child is clearly unwell or in discomfort, treatment can be started on clinical suspicion as long as two correctly collected specimens have been taken. In this instance either trimethoprim or nitrofurantoin can be chosen until the results of culture are known.

Follow-up At the end of treatment, a further urine sample should be cultured to ensure bacterial eradication.

Referral Patients with UTIs should be referred to the paediatric department for consideration of further investigation. All under five year olds will require renal imaging. Until investigations are completed the patient should remain on a prophylactic urinary antibiotic, such as trimethoprim once daily.

Haematuria

Haematuria may present as macroscopic bleeding, which is noted by parents, or as red cells seen on microscopy. All children with haematuria must be referred to the paediatric or surgical department.

UTI, abdominal or pelvic trauma, and glomerulonephritis are the most likely causes of haematuria. Red urine may sometimes be caused by eating beetroot and pink stains on an infant's nappy may be urates, but in both instances an MSU should be examined.

A history of trauma preceding the bleeding should lead to immediate referral to the surgical department and renal imaging. A concurrent history of abdominal or loin pain may indicate calculus (rare in childhood). These children should have a plain abdominal X-ray, MSU, and referral to the paediatric department.

It is important to look for oedema and to measure the blood pressure in children with haematuria. Children with oedema or hypertension must be admitted under paediatric care immediately.

If a child with haematuria is otherwise well and has no abnormal physical signs, it would be appropriate to arrange for a urea and creatinine estimation, a urine culture, and urgent referral to the next paediatric out-patient clinic.

Genital problems

- **Torsion of the testis   Balanitis   Paraphimosis
  Vulvovaginitis   Vaginal discharge   Pregnancy   Hernia**

Torsion of the testis

This urgent surgical problem is most frequent in the neonatal period and around puberty. In the older child the onset of symptoms is sometimes gradual rather than acute, with abdominal pain radiating to the groin and over the testicle. The testis is swollen, tender, and sometimes retracted. Differentiation is from epididymo-orchitis or mumps orchitis. Any boy with a painful, swollen, or discoloured testis must be referred immediately to the surgical team as early surgery may save the organ.

Balanitis

Inflammation of the prepuce is quite common in male infants and toddlers. The foreskin may become infected, causing redness and swelling. Treatment is with an oral antibiotic, such as amoxycillin or co-trimoxazole, after a swab has been taken and a urine cultured. Recurrent episodes of balanitis are an indication for surgical referral for circumcision.

Paraphimosis

Swelling of the glans penis may occur if the foreskin is irreversibly retracted. Cold compresses and lubrication may overcome the obstruction, but if they do not the child should be referred to the surgical department.

Vulvovaginitis

The symptoms of dysuria and frequency in little girls is often an indication not of a UTI but of perineal soreness. This is often associated with under- or over-hygiene of the area. The use of bubble baths may cause vulvovaginitis. A urine specimen should always be examined for infection, and it should be remembered that threadworms are a common cause of perineal irritation (see p. 202). Inspection of the vulva shows no discharge but reddened labia and introitus. The treatment is to avoid over- or under-cleansing, and to apply an emollient cream such as zinc and castor oil cream when the patient complains of discomfort. Occasionally a sore vulva may be the presentation of sexual abuse (see p. 161), but it must be remembered that a sore vulva is a common symptom in normal healthy little girls. The child's GP should be informed about the attendance.

Vaginal discharge

Causes

- Normal secretions.
- Bacterial infection for example *Streptococcus pneumoniae* and haemolytic streptococci.
- Foreign body.
- Sexual abuse (see p. 161).

The majority of pre-pubertal girls with a vaginal discharge have excessive normal secretions or a streptococcal infection. Swabs should be taken (including those for gonorrhoea and chlamydia) and the child treated with oral penicillin if streptococci are identified.

The child should be referred to the paediatric out-patient department for follow-up and further management. Identification of venereal disease warrants immediate paediatric referral.

Pregnancy

With the advent of over-the-counter pregnancy tests, the incidence of girls presenting to the A & E department with pregnancy has fallen. However, it is a condition worth remembering when adolescent girls present with vomiting or abdominal pain. Only abdominal examination must be performed. It is reasonable to ask pubertal girls with abdominal pain when their last menstrual period occurred and to sympathetically enquire whether there is a possibility of pregnancy, when appropriate. If pregnancy is confirmed, social work support should be offered and the patient's GP contacted.

Hernia

Umbilical hernias are fairly common in small babies. No treatment is indicated and the condition will usually resolve spontaneously.

Inguinal hernias are found more frequently in male babies who were born prematurely. If they are irreducible they require immediate paediatric surgical referral. The baby's legs will usually be elevated to encourage the hernia to reduce before surgery. If the hernia is reducible, urgent out-patient referral is needed.

Transilluminating scrotal swellings in infants or children are usually hydroceles and also require out-patient surgical referral. In young infants some hydroceles will disappear spontaneously.

Further reading

1. Postlethwaite, R. J. (ed.) (1986). *Clinical paediatric nephrology.* Wright, Bristol.
2. O'Donnell, B. (1985). *Abdominal pain in children.* Blackwell Scientific, Oxford.

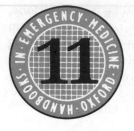

Neurology

Key points in neurology

1 Convulsions must be controlled as soon as possible, as brain damage may occur after 30 minutes convulsing.

2 Convulsions in infants may present as apnoeic spells or loss of awareness.

3 Remember the importance of hypoglycaemia in both convulsions and coma in infancy and childhood.

4 Most convulsions with a fever in children aged from six months to five years are 'febrile convulsions', but meningitis should be actively considered.

5 A high clinical awareness for the possibility of meningitis should be maintained when assessing any infant or young child who is unwell, lethargic, irritable, feverish, or vomiting.

Convulsions

- Management of convulsing child   Pharmacological control of convulsions   Further management   Causes of status epilepticus   Febrile convulsions   Convulsions in a patient known to have epilepsy   New non-febrile fits   Salaam attacks

Management of convulsing child

It is essential to clear the airway, maintain oxygenation, and stop the fit as soon as possible. While this is being done, another doctor or a nurse should obtain a rapid history from the accompany adult. The history should clarify the following points in particular.

1. How long has the child been convulsing?
2. Has the child had a recent accident, particularly involving a head injury?
3. Is he a known epileptic?
4. Has he a neurological handicap or other disease, such as diabetes?
5. Has he been unwell over the last few days? A history of increasing illness would suggest meningitis or other serious infection.
6. Could he have had access to a poisonous substance?
7. Is he on any medication? If he is on anticonvulsants, has he actually been taking them or has the dose been changed recently?

Immediate and supportive care   As soon as the patient is on the emergency trolley in a lateral position the airway should be cleared, an oral airway inserted, and a high concentration of oxygen administered through a face mask. If the child is cyanosed or breathing inadequately he should be ventilated with a bag and mask and 100 per cent oxygen. *Anaesthetic help should be requested if there is no rapid improvement.*

The patient's blood sugar should be rapidly checked with a reagent strip, such as BM Stix. If this reads less than 4 mmol/l take blood for blood sugar and insulin levels if the patient is not a diabetic. Infuse 2 ml/kg 25 per cent dextrose intravenously. A hypoglycaemic fit will then usually cease.

Pharmacological control of convulsions

Diazepam is the drug of first choice in most circumstances, and may be given intravenously or rectally. Diazemuls is the best preparation for intravenous use. It is an emulsion and is less irritant to veins than the aqueous solution. The dose for intravenous use is 0.25–0.4 mg/kg up to a maximum of 10 mg. The injection must be given slowly at a rate of not more than 2 mg/min. The injection should be stopped when the convulsion ceases (the patient often sighs), even if the full cal-culated dose has not been used. Peak brain levels occur about one minute after injection but fall to subtherapeutic levels by 15 minutes, and so fits may then recur requiring further treat-ment. Diazepam controls status epilepticus in nearly 90 per cent of cases. A second dose should be given after five min-utes if the convulsion has not ceased with the first dose of diazepam.

Problems with diazepam

1. Accidental intra-arterial injection must be avoided as this causes severe arterial spasm.

2. Too rapid injection may lead to apnoea, but this is usually brief and managed with bag-and-mask ventilation.

3. Patients who are already on a barbiturate for control of their convulsions are more likely to be apnoeic with diazepam.

4. Intramuscular injection of diazepam is ineffective and causes local tissue damage.

If intravenous access is difficult, rectal diazepam (Stesolid rectal liquid) can be given. The dose is 0.4 mg/kg. When giving Stesolid, keep the tube squeezed flat when removing it from the rectum and hold the child's buttocks together afterwards to prevent leakage of the liquid.

Do not delay in using rectal diazepam in the event of diffi-cult intravenous access. It is effective in stopping convulsions, and if the convulsion continues after a further five minutes a second dose may be given by the same route.

Note: Urgent paediatric help should be requested if the con-vulsion does not cease with the first dose of diazepam.

Use of paraldehyde If fits continue after the second dose of diazepam, paraldehyde should be used. Paraldehyde is a safe and effective drug for status epilepticus. It should be given rectally in a dose of 0.4 ml/kg diluted 50:50 with arachis oil. It is usually effective in stopping the convulsion within ten minutes.

If a child is still convulsing ten minutes after the injection of paraldehyde, preparation should be made for a phenytoin infusion if the patient is not already on this drug. Senior anaesthetic help should be requested at this stage. While the preparation is taking place, the patient's BM Stix should again be checked along with his blood pressure, pulse, and temperature. If the blood pressure has fallen, 10 ml/kg of a colloid should be infused. Active cooling measures with tepid sponging and rectal paracetamol (20 mg/kg) should be undertaken if the patient's temperature is rising. Blood should be taken for blood sugar level, acid–base status, and electrolyte levels, as metabolic abnormalities may be contributing to the resistance of the convulsions to pharmacological treatment. Raised intracranial pressure will also cause resistance of convulsions to treatment. If there are signs of raised intracranial pressure, consideration should be given to the use of intravenous mannitol. This should be done in consultation with senior paediatric staff.

Box 11.1 **Drugs for status epilepticus**

Diazepam	0.25–0.4 mg/kg intravenously
↓	0.4 mg/kg per rectum
Diazepam	0.25–0.4 mg/kg intravenously
↓	0.4 mg/kg per rectum
Paraldehyde	0.4 ml/kg in arachis oil
↓	per rectum
Phenytoin	18 mg/kg over 20–30 minutes
↓	

paralyse, ventilate, transfer to intensive care unit for thiopentone infusion

---

Administration of phenytoin ECG and blood pressure monitoring should continue while intravenous phenytoin is being given. If arrhythmias or hypotension occur, the infusion should be stopped for a few minutes and started again at a slower rate. The cardiovascular side-effects of intravenous phenytoin are result of the rate of infusion and not of the total dose infused. The initial dose of phenytoin is 18 mg/kg, and this should be given over 20–30 minutes. If the patient does not respond to this regime, he should be paralysed, ventilated, and given thiopentone in intensive care.

Box 11.2 **When to call for help**

If the *initial anticonvulsant drug* is not successful then *urgent paediatric help* should be sought immediately, although you should progress to the next stage of treatment while awaiting the paediatrician's arrival. *Failure of the second anticonvulsant drug* indicates a refractory status and *senior anaesthetic help* should be sought urgently while continuing treatment.

Further management

Once the convulsion is under control and the patient's condition is stabilized, the underlying cause must be sought. A more detailed history can be obtained and the child re-examined. Usually the paediatric team will have taken responsibility for the child at this stage. Particular note should be taken of the presence of a petechial rash (which would suggest meningococcal septicaemia), pyrexia (suggesting infection), evidence of injury, or hypertension. The neurological examination will be partially masked by the effects of the anticonvulsant drug and the post-ictal status of the patient. However, neurological signs should be sought since they may indicate an underlying focal lesion. Differences in tone and reflexes on each side of the patient, inequality of the pupils, fixed deviation of the eyes, or an abnormal doll's eye reflex will suggest an underlying focal lesion. There may be a Todd's paralysis which should resolve within 24 hours. Evidence of meningitis should be sought, although neck stiffness may be masked by the effects of the anticonvulsant.

Causes of status epilepticus

1. An atypical prolonged febrile convulsion.
2. A prolonged convulsion in a child known to have epilepsy.
3. Meningitis.
4. Trauma (head injury or hypoxia).
5. Metabolic causes, for example hypoglycaemia associated with inborn errors of metabolism and diabetes, Reye's syndrome, hypernatraemia, hyponatraemia, or poisoning.
6. Encephalitis.

Note: Sometimes patients who are in a tonic decerebrate state (usually following a severe head injury) are mistakenly thought to be in a status epilepticus. Dystonic reactions to an overdose of drugs, such as phenothiazines or metaclopramide, can also be mistaken for convulsions, but in both these conditions the rhythmic jerking characteristic of status epilepticus is absent.

Febrile convulsions

Febrile convulsions occur in 2 per cent of otherwise normal children. The majority are benign short (less than 15 minutes) grand mal convulsions triggered off by a fever in children between the ages of six months and five years.

Management In most cases the convulsion will have ceased by the time the child has arrived at the A & E department. The parents will often be very distressed. Many parents think that their child is dying when they witness a convulsion.

The child should be given paracetamol orally or, if this is not possible, rectally. Even though the convulsion has ceased and the child has recovered consciousness, the cause of the fever must be ascertained. The history and examination may provide the necessary clues. Common infections are usually the cause of febrile convulsions. These will include measles, tonsillitis, otitis media, pneumonia, and urinary tract infections. Sometimes a convulsion will occur with a diarrhoeal illness, and the organism involved is often a *Shigella* sp.

Serious consideration must be given to the possibility of meningitis in every patient with a febrile convulsion. A combination of fever and a convulsion is a common presentation for meningitis.

Referral All children presenting to an A & E department with febrile convulsions should be referred to the paediatric department. Many of these children will be admitted to hospital. This will usually include those below two years of age, those with their first febrile convulsion, those in whom meningitis is suspected or cannot be excluded clinically, and those in whom the underlying infection is not identified. Sometimes a child over two years of age who has had a previous simple febrile convulsion, in whom a clear benign source of infection has been identified, and whose parents are sensible and keen to take him home may be discharged with antipyretics by the paediatric team.

Convulsions in a patient known to have epilepsy

If the convulsion has stopped before the patient arrives at the A & E department, the patient has recovered consciousness, and examination reveals no new abnormality, admission may not be necessary. If possible, discuss the case with the patient's paediatrician or neurologist. It is advisable to take a blood sample for anticonvulsant levels and to rearrange the patient's next out-patient appointment for an earlier date.

New non-febrile fits

If a child presents with a non-febrile convulsion which has ceased before arrival at the A & E department and the child has recovered consciousness, referral should be made to the paediatric team, but admission may not be necessary. A full physical examination should be carried out, including the blood pressure and CNS. If the convulsion has been an isolated one, the child has no abnormal physical signs, and the parents are happy to take him home, he may be discharged with an EEG appointment and an urgent paediatric out-patient appointment. Before discharge, the parents should be instructed about what to do should their child have a further fit. He should be placed in the recovery position and the parents should telephone for an ambulance if the fit does not stop spontaneously within a few minutes. In the short term, bicycle riding, high gymnastic apparatus, and unsupervised swimming should be advised against.

Salaam attacks

This condition is a type of epilepsy of sudden onset in infancy. It is relatively more common in children with Down's syndrome. The episodes, which may occur many times a day, consist of sudden falling or truncal flexion, but it should be considered in any child who has serial abnormal movements of the head, trunk, or limbs. A loss of social awareness is often a feature, i.e. the baby does not seem to 'be himself'. Salaam attacks are sometimes mistaken for episodes of colic. A characteristic EEG pattern (hypsarrhythmia) is diagnostic. These infants must be admitted immediately to hospital as early treatment with ACTH will improve the prognosis for some.

Funny turns

- **Infants   Toddlers   Older children**

Children are sometimes brought to the A & E department after a parent or teacher has witnessed an alarming, but self-correcting, episode. The causes vary in differing age groups.

Infants

There are many causes for self-limiting apnoeic, cyanotic, or choking spells in babies under one year of age:

- normal shallow irregular breathing of small infant when asleep
- convulsions
- reflex laryngeal spasm with gastro-oesophageal reflux
- associated with pertussis or bronchiolitis
- perioral blueness associated with wind
- inhaled foreign body
- 'near-miss cot death' (see p. 259)
- rarely, intentional suffocation.

A good history of exactly how the episode appeared to the observer and any associated symptoms is usually very helpful. All infants with alarming episodes must be admitted for observation, some will need further investigation.

Toddlers

1. Breath-holding attacks—these episodes only occur after a toddler has been injured or thwarted. He holds his breath, rapidly turns blue, usually loses consciousness, and falls to the ground. Some children will briefly convulse. After consciousness is lost, breathing starts again and the child recovers. On examination after recovery the child is well with no abnormal physical signs. No treatment is required, but an explanation of the mechanism should be given to the child's parents.

2. Reflex anoxic episodes (pallid syncope) are episodes of vagal stimulation often occurring in the course of an illness or after an injury. The child's heart rate drops and he becomes pale, loses consciousness, and may convulse. These episodes are self-limiting and are often mistaken for

febrile convulsions. No treatment is needed, but an explanation of the mechanism should be given to the parent.

In both these attacks a good history is vital for diagnosis. Children who have had breath-holding attacks or pallid syncope do not require admission but their GP should be informed.

Older children

1. Faints—faints or vasovagal episodes often occur in school assembly. The child is described as being very pale and sweaty, and falls to the ground. Brief limb jerking is occasionally noted. On arrival at the A & E department the child has usually recovered, and on examination has no abnormal physical signs. Again, a good history is vital for the diagnosis of a vasovagal episode. If there is a poor history or the episode is unwitnessed, it may be difficult to distinguish the attack from a convulsion. If this is the case the child should be referred to the paediatrician.

Note: Episodes of syncope arising on exertion may be symptomatic of underlying obstructive congenital heart disease, such as aortic stenosis or coarctation of the aorta, or of cardiac arrythmias. In children whose syncope arises on exertion a chest X-ray and ECG should be performed and the child should be referred to the paediatric department.

2. Hyperventilation—these episodes are common in teenagers. Some upset usually triggers an episode of hyperventilation and during the attack the patient may lose consciousness. The classical physical sign of carpopedal spasm is caused by an increased arterial pH decreasing available calcium. If the patient is still hyperventilating on arrival at the A & E department, a calm environment and gentle but firm reassurance usually calms the patient down. Re-breathing into a paper bag is sometimes recommended, but is usually unnecessary.

Bacterial meningitis

- **Diagnosis of bacterial meningitis   Meningitis: treatment Meningitis: prophylaxis of contacts**

After the neonatal period, the most common cause of bacterial meningitis is *Neisseria meningitidis* (meningococcus). There is still a mortality rate of more than 5 per cent and a similar rate of permanent serious neurological sequelae. The incidence of *Haemophilus* infection has fallen following the introduction of the Hib vaccine.

Diagnosis of bacterial meningitis

Child under three years of age—bacterial meningitis is most common and yet most difficult to diagnose in its early stages in this age group. The classical signs of neck rigidity, photophobia, headache, and vomiting are often absent. A bulging fontanelle is a sign of advanced meningitis in an infant, but even this serious and late sign will be masked if the baby is dehydrated from fever and vomiting. Almost all children with meningitis have some degree of raised intracranial pressure so that, in fact, the signs and symptoms of meningitis are primarily those of raised intracranial pressure. The following are signs of possible meningitis in infants and young children:

- drowsiness (often shown by lack of eye contact with parents or doctor)
- irritability that cannot be easily soothed by parent
- poor feeding
- unexplained pyrexia
- convulsions with fever
- apnoeic or cyanotic attacks
- purpuric rash.

Older children of four years of age and over are more likely to have the classical signs of headache, vomiting, pyrexia, neck stiffness, and photophobia. In all unwell children, and children with an unexplained pyrexia, a careful search should be made for neck stiffness and a purpuric rash. The findings of such a rash in an ill child is almost pathognomic of meningococcal infection for which immediate treatment is required (see p. 34).

Meningitis: neck stiffness Neck stiffness is often a difficult sign to be sure about in an irritable child. Its absence in no way excludes meningitis in a young child. The sign is not an inability to flex the neck completely but evidence of pain, seen by watching the child's face, on neck flexion. In toddlers and older children it can be difficult to decide whether apparent neck stiffness is due to meningeal irritation or childhood resistance. Neck flexion can be made into a game by asking the child to kiss his knees, perhaps after drawing a face on it. A child who is well enough to join in a game and can kiss his knee is very unlikely to have meningitis. Kernig's and Brudzincki's signs are less helpful in childhood than neck stiffness, although they may be positive in a child who has neck rigidity.

Meningitis: referral   *Any child in whom meningitis is diagnosed or suspected must be referred urgently to the paediatrician.*

Meningitis: lumbar puncture   The purpose of a lumbar puncture is to confirm the diagnosis of meningitis and to identify the organism and its antibiotic sensitivity. Lumbar punctures should not usually be done by the A & E senior house officer. There is a risk of coning and death if a lumbar puncture is performed in a child with significantly raised intracranial pressure. Normal fundi are quite consistent with acutely severely raised intracranial pressure. The following are possible contraindications to a lumbar puncture without discussion with a senior paediatrician.

1. Focal seizures.
2. Focal neurological signs, for example asymmetry of limb movement and reflexes, ocular palsies.
3. A widespread purpuric rash in an ill child—in this case intravenous penicillin and cefotaxime should be given immediately after a blood culture.
4. Impaired conscious level—this can be rapidly assessed by judging the child's response to a peripheral painful stimulus. The normal reaction is a purposive removal of the painful stimulus. Mere withdrawal of the limb indicates a depressed conscious level.
5. Sluggish relatively dilated pupils.
6. Impaired oculocephalic reflexes (doll's eye reflexes).
7. Abnormal posture or movement—decerebrate or decorticate posturing or cycling movements of the limbs.
8. Inappropriately low pulse and elevated blood pressure.
9. Coagulation disorder.

Meningitis: treatment

If the paediatrician is unavailable and the child is very seriously ill with a purpuric rash, focal neurological signs, or a decreased conscious level, antibiotic and supportive treatment should be started after blood for culture and throat swab have been taken. A lumbar puncture should not be done as it may precipitate coning. A dose of intravenous penicillin 50 mg/kg (up to a maximum of 2 g) and cefotaxime 100 mg/kg should be given. In a case of penicillin allergy see p. 35. The antibiotics should be given slowly over 10–15 minutes. If the child is deteriorating neurologically, mannitol 0.5 g/kg can be given and the child nursed in the 30° head-up position. Consideration should be given to ventilation and the child should be transferred to intensive care. There is now evidence that dexamethasone (0.15 mg/kg) given at or before the initial antibiotic improves outcome in children with Haemophilus meningitis.

Meningitis: prophylaxis of contacts

Prophylaxis is properly the responsibility of the paediatric department and the community health team. However, following a 'meningitis scare' anxious contacts of a meningitis patient may seek advice from the A & E department. Prophylaxis with rifampicin is necessary for household contacts of a case of meningococcal meningitis. This includes everyone living in the same house as the index case. If the child was with a baby minder, the same recommendation also applies at that home. Casual or school contacts are not at risk from a sporadic case of meningococcal meningitis. Health service personnel are only at risk if they have performed mouth-to-mouth resuscitation on the patient. Prophylaxis with rifampicin is also offered to household contacts of a *Haemophilus influenzae* type B case where there is a child under four years of age in the house besides the index case. It is worth remembering that meningococcus can be isolated in the throat swabs of up to 10 per cent of the normal population. When prescribing rifampicin it is important to inform patients that it makes the contraceptive pill less effective and may turn soft contact lenses pink.

Viral meningitis

Viral meningitis is caused by mumps and enteric organisms such as Coxsackie virus and echovirus. It usually occurs in children over the age of two years. The usual signs of photophobia, headache, neck stiffness, and vomiting are present, but the child is less ill than a patient with bacterial meningitis. All such children require admission and lumbar puncture to establish the diagnosis. The virus is best isolated from faeces.

Coma

• **Causes of coma   Management**

The initial management of the child in coma can be divided into three main areas. *Immediate paediatric and, if necessary, anaesthetic aid should be requested.*

1. Maintain airway, breathing, and circulation.
2. Attempt to prevent cerebral damage, for example from hypoxia, hypotension, hypothermia, acidosis, and convulsions.
3. Diagnose and treat the treatable, for example intravenous dextrose for hypoglycaemia and intravenous antibiotics if there is any suspicion of meningitis.

Causes of coma

(Commoner causes are indicated by *italic type*.)

1. Infections with a direct cerebral effect:
   • *bacterial meningitis*
   • viral encephalitis
   • cerebral abscess.
2. Ischaemic—anoxic conditions:
   • *from fluid loss in severe gastroenteritis*
   • *from shock in overwhelming infection, for example meningococcaemia*
   • *from prolonged status epilepticus*
   • from 'near-miss cot death'

- from near drowning or hypothermia
- from heat stroke.

3. Trauma:
   - *accidental head injury with or without skull fracture*
   - *non-accidental head injury, especially in infants*
   - *shock from blood loss.*

4. Non-traumatic cerebral haemorrhage.

5. Poisoning:
   - *accidental or intentional poisoning*, for example tricyclic antidepressants, barbiturates, iron, alcohol, antifreeze, etc.
   - *drug abuse*, for example alcohol, narcotics
   - *solvent abuse.*

6. Metabolic:
   - *hypoglycaemia*, for example diabetes, severe infection, Reye's syndrome, some inborn errors of metabolism hyperinsulinaemic states
   - *hyperglycaemia and acidosis* in diabetes
   - hyperammonaemia, for example Reye's syndrome, some inborn errors of metabolism
   - uraemia and hypertension, for example haemolytic uraemic syndrome
   - hepatic failure.

Management

The patient should be admitted to the resuscitation room. Assess the airway, adequacy of respiration, and circulation clinically, treating appropriately as described in Chapter 2.

Check the patient's blood sugar by means of a Dextrostix or BM Stix test. If this is less than 4 mmol/litre, take blood for an accurate sugar level and an insulin level if the patient is not a diabetic. Then infuse 2 ml/kg of 25 per cent dextrose. In young infants with small veins 10 per cent dextrose causes less vein damage. A further BM Stix test should be performed to ensure that the hypoglycaemia is corrected. In all cases set up an intravenous infusion of 4 per cent dextrose and one-fifth normal saline or other appropriate fluid.

Monitor continuing adequacy of respiration and circulation both clinically and with a pulse oximeter, ECG, and sphygmo-manometer (both manual and automatic).

If there is any possibility of opiate poisoning the patient should have a trial of naloxone.

A history should be taken from the accompanying adult or ambulance attendant, including whether the patient is known to have a chronic disease, such as diabetes or epilepsy, whether there has been any recent injury or access to poisons, and the history of the patient's health in the last 24 hours.

Examine the patient, looking for external signs of trauma (particularly to the head), a rash, (particularly a purpuric rash), focal neurological signs, jaundice, hypertension, or enlarged liver or spleen. The fundi should be carefully examined for papilloedema or retinal haemorrhages. The oculomotor reflexes should be tested. Absent 'doll's eye' reflex in an unconscious patient suggests brain-stem dysfunction. Posture should be examined by looking for decorticate or decerebrate postures. The pupils should be examined for size, reactivity, and equality.

An assessment of the depth of coma should be performed using a coma scale (see p. 61). If the Glasgow coma scale is less than 8, an anaesthetist should be summoned. The patient will require intubation to protect the airway.

It is important to keep the patient normothermic, normotensive, normoglycaemic, well oxygenated, and in normal acid–base balance to prevent secondary brain damage. Initial investigations should include a blood sugar and arterial blood gas estimations, haemoglobin and blood smear, electrolyte levels, and blood culture.

Further investigations will be ordered by the paediatrician, depending on the history and clinical findings. Lumbar puncture should not be performed, because of the risk of coning, until raised intracranial pressure has been excluded, and after a CT scan. If there are signs of increasing intracranial pressure (see p. 61), hyperventilation and intravenous mannitol may be needed.

If there is any suggestion of bacterial meningitis or the condition cannot be excluded, intravenous penicillin and cefotaxime should be given (see p. 35). If viral encephalitis is thought likely, intravenous acylovir should be given.

Arrangements may be needed for the patient to undergo a CT scan and to be transferred to a paediatric intensive care unit. For transfer requirements, see p. 66.

Occasionally, a patient, usually a teenager, will be 'shamming' unconsciousness. The absence of any genuine physical signs usually makes this obvious. Counselling for an underlying behaviour problem may be required.

Headache

Headache is often a feature of acute upper respiratory infections, and a worried parent may bring a child to the A & E department because of concern about meningitis. It is usually not difficult to differentiate meningitis from other infectious illnesses in the child old enough to complain of a headache. If in doubt, of course, referral to the paediatrician would be appropriate.

Headache can be caused by referred pain from dental disease or sinusitis. The latter is uncommon in young children as the frontal sinuses are not well developed until about 10 years of age. Headache may be associated with systemic hypertension, and all children presenting with headache must have their blood pressure measured. Bleeding from an arteriovenous malformation is a rare event in childhood. It may present as the sudden onset of a very severe headache. Loss of consciousness and stiff neck are less common than in adults. Children will usually show, in addition to the headache, a seizure, focal neurological deficit, or general increased irritability.

A child with recurrent headache may also present to the A & E department when parents are distressed with the child's symptom and worried about possible underlying causes. A full history and careful examination is necessary, including the blood pressure.

Migraine and recurrent stress headaches are common in middle childhood. Migraine is typically associated with nausea and vomiting and is relieved by sleep. A few children with migraine have temporary neurological abnormalities, such as hemiplegia. These children must be admitted for investigation. A child with a headache present on waking or one whose headache wakens him from sleep should be referred to the paediatric department as this may be a sign of raised intracranial pressure.

A child with an uncomplicated recurrent headache should be referred back to his GP after reassurance to the parents that there is nothing acutely wrong.

Acute motor weakness

• Guillain–Barré syndrome   Bell's palsy

Guillain–Barré syndrome

Guillain–Barré syndrome is now the most common form of acute motor weakness in childhood. This illness usually occurs after a mild viral infection. Patients are sometimes thought to be hysterical when they first present. The development of peripheral nerve weakness usually starts in the legs and the patient often complains of a painful back. The reflexes are depressed and there may be painful paraesthesiae. Later on, bulbar signs, dysphonia, and dysphasia may develop. All patients with Guillain–Barré syndrome must be admitted under paediatric care. Some will progress to ventilatory failure as the intercostal muscles are involved.

Bell's palsy

The sudden onset of unilateral facial weakness involving all three branches of the facial nerve is not uncommon in children. Parents are often very alarmed by this and may bring the child straight to an A & E department thinking that he has had a stroke. Children with facial weakness should be referred to the paediatrician for assessment although they may be managed as an out-patient.

Bell's palsy is a diagnosis of exclusion, and so a careful examination for other neurological signs should be made. Additional signs would indicate a possible underlying tumour as the cause of the abnormality. The blood pressure should be measured as hypertension in childhood occasionally presents as isolated nerve palsies. The presence of a vesicular rash suggests the Ramsey–Hunt syndrome, and an erythematous or indurated rash suggests Lyme disease (for which penicillin or erythromycin would be beneficial). Evidence of local inflammation in the ear or mastoids should be sought.

In Bell's palsy, complete recovery is usual in over 90 per cent of children in six to eight weeks. If the child is seen in the first two or three days a five-day course of prednisone, 2 mg/kg/day in two daily doses, is often prescribed, although there is no proof of efficacy. An eye patch and chloramphenicol eye ointment should be used in patients who cannot close the eye properly in order to prevent conjunctival infection and damage. Occasionally there is poor recovery, and cosmetic surgery may be required later.

Further reading

1. Gordon, N. and McKinley, I. (ed.) (1986). *Neurologically sick children: treatment and management.* Blackwell Scientific, Oxford.
2. Levin, N. and Heyderman, R. S. (1991). Bacterial meningitis. In *Recent advances in paediatrics*, Vol. 9 (ed. T. J. David), pp. 1–19. Churchill Livingstone, Edinburgh.

CHAPTER 12

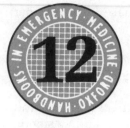

Skin and infectious diseases

Presentation of skin diseases

Children may be brought to the A & E department because of the sudden appearance, or worsening, of a rash or its poor response to treatment.

The diagnosis of a rash is based on its history, appearance, distribution, and associated physical signs. An ophthalmoscope set at about 8 dioptres is often helpful for close inspection of skin lesions.

1. Erythematous maculopapular rashes are usually due to an infectious disease or an allergic reaction.

2. Itchy skin lesions suggest eczema, scabies, or insect bites.

3. Vesicobullous eruptions are characteristic of chickenpox, herpes simplex, and hand, foot, and mouth disease. Staphylococcal infection, bullous erythema multiforme, and drug reactions are less common but potentially more serious causes of a vesicobullous rash.

4. A sore mouth may be due to primary herpes simplex, candida infection, scarlet fever, or rarer more serious diseases such as Stevens–Johnson syndrome or Kawasaki's disease.

5. A non-itchy scaly lesion suggests psoriasis or a fungal infection.

6. Purpuric (non-blanching) lesions are caused by vasculitis, trauma, or clotting disorders, and always require paediatric referral.

Note: A purpuric rash in an ill child is almost certainly meningococcal septicaemia. Urgent treatment is needed (p. 35).

Eczema

Sudden deterioration in eczema is usually due to infection. Bacterial infection causes pustules, discharge, and crusting. The causative organisms are usually *Staphylococcus aureus* and beta haemolytic streptococci. For one or two small infected areas a topical antiseptic, such as 10 per cent providone–iodine cream, or an antiseptic hydrocortisone cream, such as Vioform HC, may be sufficient. Topical antibiotics are best avoided as they can cause sensitization. Any more widespread infection requires oral penicillin and flucloxacillin for 7–14 days.

Ill or pyrexial children with widespread infection should be admitted to hospital, but others can be treated as out-patients. A skin swab is important to ensure that the organism is sensitive to the antibiotics prescribed. Most children with infected eczema will noticeably improve within 48 hours and they should be reviewed then. If they have not improved by then, the usual explanations are non-compliance with treatment or bacterial resistance, or else the infection is due to herpes virus. The child should be referred to the paediatric department.

Primary herpes simplex infection may cause serious systemic illness in eczematous children. Vesicles can appear over the face, trunk, and limbs, and they soon turn to umbilicated pustules. Scratching and secondary infection may make herpes infection difficult to distinguish from simple bacterial infection. The virus can be identified by culture of skin exudate or, more rapidly, by examination of vesicular fluid under the electron microscope. Mild cases are self-limiting, but severe cases with systemic illness and fever require treatment with antibiotics and intravenous acyclovir.

If the eczema is not infected but help is sought because of itching, an emollient, such as emulsifying ointment or white soft paraffin, can be used whenever the skin is dry. If night-time itching is disturbing the child, the sedative effect of Vallergan (trimeprazine) tablets may reduce the damaging effect of scratching. These children should be referred back to their GP for continued management.

Seborrhoeic dermatitis

Seborrhoeic dermatitis is most easily recognized by the thick scalp scale known as 'cradle cap'. On the face, neck, and in the nappy area the rash is greasy, red, and scaly, but apparently not itchy. The application of a mild keratolytic agent such as 1 per cent salicylic acid in white soft paraffin twice a week, followed 12 hours later by shampooing, will treat the cradle cap, and 1 per cent hydrocortisone ointment is suitable for other areas. The child should be referred back to his GP.

Psoriasis

A guttate psoriasis with round red scaly lesions over the trunk may follow a streptococcal throat infection. Less frequently, children present with typical red and scaly psoriatic lesions on the extensor aspects of the elbows and knees, and in the scalp. Skin and scalp should be treated with coal tar ointment or shampoo. Failing improvement with coal tar, 0.1 per cent dithranol ointment can be prescribed. Steroid creams should be avoided as their use is associated with early relapse of the skin condition. Refer the patient back to his GP.

Infestations and infections

- **Scabies   Fungal infection—tinea   Warts   Molluscum contagiosum   Impetigo**

Scabies

The cause of scabies is infestation with the mite *Sarcopes scabiei.* There is a widespread papular urticarial rash on the trunk and limbs. It is often most noticeable on the feet and ankles in toddlers. Scratch marks are often seen, but burrows can be difficult to find. Scabies is characterized by severe itching of the skin, particularly at night. If other family members are also itching, the diagnosis is very clear. There is a one-month latent period from infestation to the allergic urticarial rash.

Treatment is with 1 per cent lindane lotion which should be applied to all skin from the neck downwards and left for 24 hours before bathing off. For children under five, very thin individuals, and epileptics, aqueous malathion should be used. If using malathion, the treatment should be repeated three days later. All bed clothes and clothing should be washed. The rest of the family should be advised to seek advice from their GP as they may also be affected.

Fungal infection—tinea

Tinea corporis produces round red scaly non-itchy lesions which are sometimes mistaken for psoriasis. The classical paler centre which gives the lesion its name of ringworm appears later in the disease. The lesions should be treated with clotrimazole (1 per cent) or miconazole (2 per cent) cream twice daily. Treatment is usually required for two or three weeks and should be continued for several days after the lesions have disappeared.

Tinea unguum appears as a thickened and yellow nail not caused by trauma, or as a persistent or relapsing paronychia. A nail paring can be examined by the microbiology laboratory for hyphae. *Tinea capitum* presents as bald patches from which broken hairs protrude. The hair is fluorescent under Wood's light. Both nail and scalp infections are difficult to treat and require systemic griseofulvin. These patients should be referred back to their GP or to a dermatologist for treatment since long-term follow-up is required.

Warts

Warts and plantar warts (verrucae) are virus-induced hyper-keratotic skin tumours. Verrucae are sometimes presented as foreign bodies in the foot. Warts are self-limiting but disfiguring, and in the case of verrucae are often painful. Treatment is either time consuming (keratolytic) or painful (destructive methods, such as freezing and currettage). Children should be advised to await resolution or be referred back to the GP.

Molluscum contagiosum

Molluscum contagiosum is another virus-induced skin infection. The rash consists of pearly papules with a central umbilication in crops often around the face, axillae, neck, and knees. The papules will disappear spontaneously but this may take several months. Their disappearance can be speeded up by breaking the skin with a needle and extruding the caseous contents. The child should be referred back to his GP.

Impetigo

Impetigo is a staphylococcal or streptococcal infection of the skin which develops on skin damaged by abrasion, insect bites, scabies, or other preceding skin injury. The initial pustules soon rupture and leave a yellow crust over a weeping red area. Small lesions can be treated by cleansing and an antiseptic cream such as 10 per cent povidone–iodine. Widespread lesions warrant systemic flucloxacillan for a week. A swab should be taken first to make sure that the organism is sensitive to the antibiotic prescribed.

Allergic rashes

• **Urticaria   Angioneurotic oedema   Insect bites**

Urticaria

The sudden onset of urticaria ('nettle rash') is common. Sometimes a precipitating factor is identified in a child known to be allergic to foodstuffs such as egg, nuts, or fish. More frequently, no allergen is identified. Treatment with oral antihistamines is usually effective.

Angioneurotic oedema

A few children with an allergic reaction will have swelling of the face, including the lips and sometimes the tongue and buccal mucosa. These children should be referred to the paediatrician as there is a small risk of laryngeal oedema.

Insect bites

Insect bites present as multiple itching papules with urticaria. Usually they are in crops on the trunk and limbs. There may be no history of exposure to insect bites, particularly in young children. Topical antihistamines are not effective. Calamine lotion or crotamiton (10 per cent cream or lotion) are mildly antipruritic and may help symptomatically. Any pets at home should be treated with an insecticide.

Nappy rash

A rash in the nappy area is usually ammoniacal dermatitis with red ulcerated areas but with sparing of the inside of skin folds. It is best treated by leaving the nappy off until the rash has healed. (This may take two or three days.) Its return can be prevented by frequent nappy changes, cleansing, and a barrier cream. A rash which causes red macerated skin inside the groin folds and satellite areas on the abdomen is caused by *Candida* and requires topical nystatin cream. The skin of babies with eczema or seborrhoeic dermatitis who have nappy area involvement may improve with an anti-fungal and hydrocortisone cream such as Nystaform or Canesten HC.

Painful mouths

1. *Candida* infection of the buccal mucosa is common in babies up to a few weeks old. The baby may cry on sucking or refuse feeds, although he is otherwise well. White patches with a red base are seen in the mouth. Treatment is with oral nystatin after feeds.

2. The most common cause of stomatitis in young children is *primary* herpes simplex. This unpleasant disease starts abruptly with a painful ulcerated mouth, fever, and refusal to eat. Treatment is symptomatic with analgesics. Solid foods cannot be attempted for several days, but most

children can be managed at home with drinks of milk through a straw. A few children may need admitting for nursing care if the parents cannot be relied upon to prevent dehydration.

3. Coxsackie virus A16 is the usual cause of hand, foot, and mouth disease. The mouth lesions are ulcers, but vesicles are seen on the palms and dorsal surfaces of the hands and sometimes on the feet. No treatment is needed.

4. Stevens–Johnson syndrome is a potentially fatal disorder which presents with mouth ulcers in conjunction with a vesicular or bullous erythema multiforme which may be present on the perineum. The condition is sometimes precipitated by drugs (particularly sulphonamides) or may occur following an upper respiratory tract infection. Special hazards are a severe conjunctivitis, which may lead to blindness, and septicaemia from secondary infection of affected skin with Gram-negative organisms. Any child suspected of having Stevens–Johnson syndrome must be admitted to hospital under paediatric and ophthalmic care.

Purpura

Purpura is a red or purple skin rash that does not blanch on pressure, which is brought about by blood in the skin. Causes include vasculitis, thrombocytopenia, a clotting disorder, or trauma. All children with purpura should be referred to the paediatrician.

1. *A purpuric rash in an ill child is usually meningococcal septicaemia and is a medical emergency* (see p. 35).

2. Idiopathic thrombocytopenic purpura is the most common cause of a low platelet count in childhood. The disease often appears to be initiated by a preceding minor infection. Purpura may be found in any site but is often seen as large ecchymoses over those sites that children commonly bruise and also as petechiae on the trunk. In most cases the disease is self-limiting. Intracranial bleeding rarely occurs but can be fatal.

3. Drugs, particularly sulphonamides, can cause thrombocytopenia and present as purpura.

4. Leukaemia is a less common but important disease to consider in patients with purpura. Other features to look for are a short history of tiredness, pallor, or limb pain. Hepatosplenomegaly may be found on abdominal examination.

5. Henoch–Schonlein purpura is the most common non-thrombocytopenic purpura. There is a vasculitis of unknown aetiology. The earlier skin lesions blanch but soon become purpuric. The purpura is almost always on the lower limbs and there is accompanying oedema which may be quite marked in the scrotum. Another feature is arthritis affecting large joints, such as the knees and ankles. Most children have microscopic haematuria and in some this is macroscopic. A few children with Henoch–Schonlein purpura have nephritis and so the blood pressure must be checked. Abdominal pain is a common complaint and some children pass blood per rectum. There is no specific treatment. All children should be referred to the paediatrician but milder cases may be managed by them as outpatients.

6. Bruises, particularly in different stages of discoloration may be caused by child abuse (p. 152).

7. The haemophilic patient should be managed as described on p. 240.

Common infectious diseases of childhood

• **Risk groups**

Risk groups

Certain groups of children may be at serious risk from the common infectious diseases of childhood. Children with immune deficiency syndromes or those on immune suppressant drugs should be referred to the paediatric department, or advice should be sought from their specialist if they present with an infectious disease or have been in contact with one. Children with cystic fibrosis can be seriously ill with measles, whooping cough, or chickenpox, and should be referred if they have one of these diseases or have been in contact with one of them.

Neonates are generally immune to the common exanthems of childhood as they have antibodies from their mothers, but if they do develop one of these diseases they may be seriously ill. Chickenpox is a special risk in this age group. Neonates with an exanthem should be referred to the paediatric team.

Measles (rubeola) This has a characteristic prodromal phase of fever, coryza, conjunctivitis, and a cough. The diagnosis is made at this stage by seeing Koplick's spots—white dots on a red background—on the inside of the cheeks. When the exanthem appears the child's fever rises further as a macular rash starts behind the ears and spreads, becoming papular, over the face, arms, and trunk. Some children have otitis media, pneumonia, or diarrhoea and vomiting. Encephalitis is rare but potentially fatal. Measles can still occur mildly if a child has received measles vaccine. Admission is rarely necessary for a child with measles unless he is very sick or has underlying chronic disease. Infectivity continues for five days after the rash has appeared, and the incubation period is two weeks.

German measles (rubella) Rubella is a much milder infection than measles and its chief health impact is in congenital rubella. The rash is maculopapular, on the face and trunk, and usually disappears over a day or so. Posterior cervical and occipital lymphadenopathy is characteristic. The incubation period of rubella is 14–21 days and infectivity continues until the rash has gone. In older children a transient arthralgia or arthritis occurs occasionally. Treatment is symptomatic.

Roseola infantum This is characterized by a fever with no apparent cause which subsides as a maculopapular rash appears over the trunk and arms, fading within 24 hours. No treatment is required.

Erythema infectiosum or slapped cheek disease The causative agent in this disease is parvovirus B19. The rash begins with bright red cheeks and circumoral pallor. It then appears over the limbs in a confluent or reticular pattern. The disease is self-limiting and benign. In older children arthralgia may occur. In patients with a haemolytic anaemia, such as sickle cell disease or thalassaemia, parvovirus may precipitate an aplastic crisis (p. 239).

Scarlet fever—see p. 170.

Chickenpox   Chickenpox produces successive crops of itchy vesicles on a red base on the face, scalp, and trunk. Lesions may occur in the mouth, genitalia, or eyes. Treatment is symptomatic, but chloramphenicol or gentamycin ointment may be used for the eyes as secondary bacterial infection is likely. Complications are uncommon in children, but occasionally a chickenpox pneumonitis occurs for which intravenous acyclovir is used. The disease is infectious from 24 hours before the rash appears until the last crop of vesicles has scabbed.

Other viruses (such as echoviruses and adenoviruses)   These can produce a measles- or German-measles-like rash in association with fever and upper respiratory tract or gastrointestinal symptoms. Treatment is symptomatic.

Mumps   Mumps causes pain and swelling in one or both parotid glands. The swelling is often easier to see than palpate. The angle of the mandible is obscured and the earlobe is pushed upward and outward. This is most clearly seen if the patient is observed from the back. In the mouth, redness and swelling can be seen around the parotid duct. Mumps meningitis is quite common during this condition and is the most common cause of aseptic meningitis. Orchitis is uncommon in childhood. If it is suspected, torsion of the testicle should also be considered as a cause of the testicular pain and swelling. Patients with mumps are infectious until the parotid swelling has subsided, and the incubation period is 14–24 days.

Hepatitis A   Many infections with hepatitis A are anicteric and pass undiagnosed. The prodromal illness consists of fever, malaise, anorexia, and nausea. Jaundice, dark urine, or pale stools are usually the cause for A & E attendance. No treatment is required for children with hepatitis A, but they should be referred to their GP to be supervised until the jaundice has subsided. Hepatitis A immunoglobulin is not routinely recommended for contacts but should be considered for pregnant mothers and any contact who is chronically ill.

Eye infections

• Conjunctivitis Periorbital cellulitis

Conjunctivitis (for neonatal conjunctivitis see p. 250)

Red, painful, or purulent conjunctivae, without preceding trauma may be infected with *Haemophilus influenzae*, streptococci or staphylococci, or a virus. Some cases of conjunctivitis occur in the course of a systemic viral infection with measles or adenovirus.

Treatment, after a swab for bacterial culture has been taken, is by cleansing the eye with damp cotton wool followed by the installation of chloramphenicol eye drops every two hours while the child is awake, and chloramphenicol eye ointment at night. Tetracycline eye ointment every six hours is an alternative. Two-hourly treatment is usually necessary for only a day or so then after which every six to eight hours will suffice.

Recurrent watery eye is common in infancy and is due to a blocked tear duct. Most improve spontaneously.

Non-infective causes of conjunctivitis include reaction to eye drops already being used, chemical irritation from chlorine in swimming pools, and allergic conjunctivitis. The latter may demonstrate striking conjunctival oedema. Systemic or topical antihistamines may help, but the reaction is usually self-limiting. Occasionally, conjunctivitis is seen as part of a systemic illness such as Stevens–Johnson syndrome (p. 232) or Kawasaki's disease (p. 237).

Periorbital cellulitis

This is a serious infection which can lead to eye damage cavernous sinus thrombosis, or meningitis.

The child has pain and swelling around the eye and in the eyelid. He is often unwell or pyrexial, but if he is not the condition can be mistaken for conjunctivitis. However, the inflammation is more obvious in the periorbital tissues than in the conjunctivae.

The child should be admitted for intravenous antibiotics effective against staphylococci, streptococci, and *Haemophilus influenzae*.

Kawasaki's disease

This is an uncommon vasculitic disease of unknown aetiology. It is important to recognize, as early diagnosis and treatment in hospital (human immunoglobulin intravenously and oral aspirin) can reduce the risk of late serious sequelae (coronary artery aneurysm and death).

The diagnosis is considered in a patient who has some, or all, of the following features:

- prolonged (more than five days) fever with no apparent cause
- non-purulent conjunctivitis
- cutaneous rash (usually urticarial)
- dry fissured lips
- red tongue with enlarged papillae
- peeling fingers
- lymph gland enlargement
- arthralgia
- thrombocytosis

Such patients should be referred to the paediatrician.

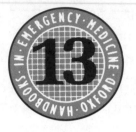

CHAPTER 13

Blood disorders

Blood disorders

Children with a haemoglobinopathy may develop acute symptoms from their disease or need A & E treatment for another related problem, such as trauma.

Sickle cell anaemia

- Infection in sickle cell patients Sickle cell crises
  Anaesthesia in sickle cell patients

Infection in sickle cell patients

Infection is frequently due to pneumococcal disease associated with defective splenic function even in the presence of a large or normal spleen. A seriously ill sickle cell patient probably has pneumococcal or salmonella septicaemia. Urgent paediatric help should be requested and intravenous penicillin or ampicillin given.

Sickle cell crises

Painful crises may occur in any site. They are easily confused with, and may coexist with, acute infection.

1. Abdominal pain due to sickling in abdominal blood vessels may suggest appendicitis or cholecystitis.

238

2. Limb sickling may mimic osteomyelitis or acute arthritis.
3. Chest pain and dyspnoea may mimic pneumonia but be due to the acute chest syndrome.
4. Small children develop swelling of the hands and fingers resembling tuberculous dactylitis but with a more acute onset.

Patients should be referred to the paediatrician.

In the treatment of acute episodes it is sensible to assume that infection is present and to give antibiotic cover. In view of the frequency of pneumococcal infection, a penicillin should be used. Erythromycin may be used in the penicillin-sensitive patient. Sickle cell patients frequently have impaired renal concentrating ability and dehydrate rapidly, which makes their symptoms worse. Ample fluid replacement, intravenously if necessary, must be the rule. Dextrans and other colloids offer no advance over 4 per cent dextrose and 0.18 per cent saline. Crises may be very painful and demoralizing for patients prone to recurrent attacks. Analgesics must be given regularly and in sufficient dosage to remove pain.

Anaesthesia in sickle cell patients

Anaesthesia in any child with haemoglobin S, including any child with sickle cell trait, needs to be performed with care to ensure good oxygenation and to avoid acidosis. The anaesthetist should always be informed in advance if operation is contemplated. Oxygen is given post-operatively until the child has fully recovered from the effects of the anaesthetic.

Sickle tests should be available to every A & E department and should be used to screen any child of Afro-Caribbean origin with a painful condition or who needs an anaesthetic. A sickle test will not distinguish sickle cell disease from sickle cell trait, but patients with sickle cell anaemia can usually be recognized by their low haemoglobin.

Thalassaemia

Thalassaemia major causes a severe haemolytic anaemia with marked hepatosplenomegaly. Lifelong blood transfusion is necessary every few weeks. This leads to iron overload which is treated with regular subcutaneous injections of desferrioxamine, given at home most nights with a battery-powered syringe driver. Some patients develop local erythema at the site of injection but these usually recover spontaneously.

Complications which may develop in thalassaemia major and present to the A & E department include the following.

1. Overwhelming bacterial sepsis due to splenectomy or a non-functioning spleen. Blood culture should be performed and high-dose intravenous penicillin or ampicillin given.

2. Infection with *Yersinia enterocolitica* whose growth is encouraged by the iron overload.

3. Cardiac arrhythmias in older patients with iron overload.

4. Endocrine disorders due to fibrosis secondary to iron overload. These include diabetes mellitus and hypocalcaemia due to fibrosis of the parathyroids.

Patients who have received blood transfusions outside Europe should be regarded as high-risk cases for hepatitis B and possibly HIV infection. Gloves should be worn when their blood is collected. Samples should be labelled with a 'Risk of Infection' label.

Glucose-6-phosphate dehydrogenase deficiency (G-6-PD)

Patients with a G-6-PD deficiency usually come from Africa, Asia, and Southern Europe. The importance of the condition in the A & E department is that certain drugs can precipitate episodes of haemolysis. Aspirin, nitrofurantoin, and sulphonamides (including co-trimoxazole) may cause haemolysis and should be avoided in patients with G-6-PD deficiency.

Management of the haemophiliac patient

The haemophilias include classical haemophilia (haemophilia A) due to factor VIII deficiency, Christmas disease (haemophilia B) due to factor IX deficiency, and von Willebrand's disease (haemophilia C) due to a defect of the von Willebrand factor, of which factor VIII forms a part. The two former are inherited in a sex-linked manner, the latter is autosomal with both dominant and recessive patterns.

The symptoms of classical haemophilia and Christmas disease are identical, and the two diseases can only be distinguished by blood tests.

However, as different clotting factor concentrates are used in their treatment, an accurate diagnosis is essential. Affected patients should be registered at a haemophilia centre and issued with a green card giving details of their disorder. In cases of difficulty the haemophilia centre should be able to give advice about precise diagnosis and the usual treatment. Affected boys bruise easily, and superficial bruises rarely need treatment. Ice-packs applied early will often help a more severe bruise to settle.

Bleeding into joints is the major problem with both diseases. The large joints are usually involved, particularly knees, ankles, and elbows. Early treatment by clotting factor replacement is the rule, in order to prevent joint damage and late osteoarthritis. Affected patients are often able to identify a joint bleed at a very early stage, well before any objective signs are visible or palpable for the doctor unfamiliar with haemophilia. It is unusual for undiagnosed haemophiliacs to present for the first time in an A & E department, and so most will be visitors unfamiliar with the local haemophilia centre, patients on home treatment who have used up their supplies, or patients with mild disease who do not normally attend a haemophilia centre. In all cases, do not hesitate to ask the patient or parent what treatment is usually given, which vein is preferred for injection, and what other treatment is needed. These patients usually know a lot about their own disease and it is common sense to pay attention to their views.

Most joint bleeds respond to a dose of clotting factor which brings the blood level up to 20–30 per cent. Bleeds are usually spontaneous and 80 per cent settle with one injection. Bleeds due to injury need higher doses which may need to be repeated, and the patient should be referred to the local haemophilia centre as soon as possible. The joint may be more comfortable if a crepe bandage is applied. For severe bleeds a plaster of Paris backslab or Robert Jones bandage may be helpful. Plaster should never be applied all around the limb in case further bleeding causes vascular obstruction, and any plaster cylinder should be split. Joint aspiration is rarely necessary, but will relieve pressure, and hence pain, in severe haemarthrosis with a large hot tense joint. It must be undertaken with full sterile precautions and further clotting factor subsequently given in an attempt to prevent further bleeding. Aspiration of joints should not usually be carried out by A & E staff.

The dose of clotting factor needed is calculated as follows:

$$\text{Factor dose needed (ml)} = \frac{\text{Weight (kg)} \times \% \text{ rise needed}}{\text{constant } (k)}$$

where $k = 1.5$ for factor VIII and $k = 0.9$ for factor IX.

Other bleeds or suspected bleeds which require clotting factor treatment include head injury, bleeding in the floor of the mouth and the neck which could obstruct respiration, and bleeding in the perineum which could obstruct the urethra. Cerebral haemorrhage comes high on the list of causes of death in haemophilia. Affected patients should be given a dose of clotting factor calculated to bring the blood level up to at least 80 per cent immediately and the patient admitted for observation. A CT scan should be arranged urgently and the neurosurgical team and haemophilia centre contacted at once. Haematomas can be removed and patients may make a full recovery.

Other bleeding complications include bleeding from the mouth and gums, and epistaxis. They can sometimes be stopped by local application of a 50:50 mixture of topical thrombin and 1:1000 adrenalin, but recurrent and resistant bleeds need factor replacement to a level of around 25 per cent, which may need to be repeated until the lesion has healed. Tranexamic acid (Cyclokapron) is helpful for bleeds from the mouth and gastrointestinal tract, but not for joint bleeds. The dose is 250 mg per 10 kg body weight three times daily; both tablets and an elixir are available. Patients with von Willebrand's disease tend to be less severely affected than those with haemophilia A and B. However, some patients are severely affected, behaving like severe haemophiliac boys. In addition, severely affected adolescent girls may have bad menorrhagia. Joint bleeds may be painful and need analgesia. Paracetamol may be ineffective, and mixtures of paracetamol and codeine are better. Mefenamic acid is often helpful (25 mg/kg/day in three divided doses). Fractures are relatively common in haemophiliacs. Bone rarefaction from disuse and inflammation may be a predisposing factor. Fortunately they heal well. Clotting factor replacement for several days is usually recommended. Remember that any plaster should be split. The only exception to this is for a patient who is under continuous observation in hospital, when the distal part of the limb can be observed for circulatory or neurological impairment.

Any laceration large enough to need suturing will need high-dose clotting factor replacement daily until the wound has healed. The blood level needs to be maintained above 50 per cent throughout this time. Wounds heal slowly in haemophiliacs, and even small cuts will break down with the formation of loose jelly-like clots and risk of infection unless covered by replacement treatment. Do not be misled by the fact that the wound has clotted well after suturing; it may break down and bleed up to several days later. When possible, it is sensible to use adhesive strips rather than stitches to bring wound edges together.

Normal immunization can be given in haemophiliacs, but they are better given subcutaneously rather than intramuscularly. Tetanus prophylaxis should not be omitted because of haemophilia.

Bleeding after dental extraction calls for clotting factor replacement. Tranexamic acid is often helpful. Oral penicillin V may help to prevent bleeding by depressing growth of oral of oral bacteria which may provoke fibrinolysis. Bleeding from the site of desquamating or recently desquamated primary teeth may be stopped by local pressure and/or topical thrombin and adrenalin (see above).

Haemophiliacs born before 1985 who have been treated with clotting factor concentrates may be infected with HIV or hepatitis B. The products now used are safe, and so there is virtually no risk that younger haemophiliacs will have contracted these infections. However, if there is any doubt, it is sensible to treat a haemophiliac patient as potentially infectious. Collect blood samples, treat lacerations, and give injections wearing gloves, and label blood samples with a 'Risk of Infection' warning.

CHAPTER 14

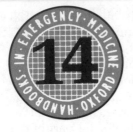

Neonatal problems

Neonatal resuscitation

- **Resuscitation management   Action to take if poor
  response to resuscitation   When to stop resuscitation
  Post-resuscitation care**

Occasionally an asphyxiated baby, newly born in an ambulance or at home, may be brought to the A & E department for
resuscitation. A baby who is born quickly and unexpectedly
and is asphyxiated is very likely to be a preterm baby. Staff in
the A & E department should be able to resuscitate such an
infant before transferring him to the special care baby unit or
neonatal intensive care unit.

The equipment and drugs detailed in Tables 14.1, 14.2, and

Table 14.1 • Equipment for neonatal airway and breathing
management

1. Neonatal face mask for oxygen delivery
2. Suction catheter with a soft tip (maximum pressure of 100 mmHG
    on the suction machine)
3. Infant oral airways sizes 000–1
4. Laerdal infant bag and mask
5. Two straight-bladed neonatal laryngoscopes
6. Endotracheal tubes: sizes 2.5, 3.0, and 3.5 mm
7. A cold fibre optic light source (optional)
8. Chest drain set

Table 14.2 • Equipment for umbilical vein catheterization

1. Scalpel
2. Fine sterile feeding tube
3. A pair of untoothed forceps
4. Umbilical tape
5. Silk stitch
6. Adhesive tape suitable for delicate skin

Table 14.3 • Drugs for neonatal resuscitation

Drugs	Dose	Route
Sodium bicarbonate, 8.4%	1–2 mmol/kg	IV
Dextrose, 10%	2 ml/kg	IV
Naloxone	10 µg/kg	IM or IV
Adrenalin, 1:10 000	0.1 ml/kg	IV or IT
Atropine	0.02 mg/kg	IV
Calcium chloride, 10%	0.5 ml/kg (slowly)	IV
Frusemide	1–2 mg/kg	IV

14.3 will be required for neonatal resuscitation. Some of this will be standard A & E equipment.

Resuscitation management

The infant's colour, respiratory effort and rate, and pulse rate should be assessed.

Paediatric help should be summoned immediately, but the initial resuscitation should be commenced while awaiting the paediatrician.

1. If the baby is pink, active, and crying vigorously, no active resuscitation is required. The baby should be dried and kept warm with warmed blankets and an improvised hat made from Tubigrip. Unless the oropharynx is full of meconium or maternal blood, the baby should not be routinely sucked out as this may cause reflex vagal bradycardia and apnoea. If the mother is well enough, the baby should be kept with her. If she is unwell or receiving treatment she should be shown the baby so that she can be reassured that he is well.

The baby should be under observation until transferred to the post-natal ward or special care baby unit. If the infant is less than 2 kg, or cold, or unwell, a BM Stix should be checked. Hypoglycaemia (2 mmol or less) should be urgently confirmed with a venous sample of blood. A hypoglycaemic baby should be fed if asymptomatic or given 10 per cent dextrose (2 ml/kg as a bolus initially) intravenously if he is jittery or convulsing. The feed should be 15–30 ml of a baby milk, but if none is available in the A & E department 10 per cent dextrose will be adequate. Treatment of hypoglycaemia must be immediate and a further BM Stix checked to assess response.

2. If the baby is blue and apnoeic, or gasping, with a heart rate of 100 or above and the tone only slightly decreased, he may respond to peripheral stimulation and facial oxygen or ventilation by bag and mask with oxygen. However, if there is no spontaneous respiration within one minute, or the heart rate starts to fall, the baby should be intubated by the oral route. A size 3 endotracheal tube is preferred, but below 28 weeks a size 2.5 tube may be needed. If the mother has had an opiate during labour, the baby may become pink but not start breathing spontaneously. Under these circumstances intravenous or intramuscular naloxone (10 μg/kg) should be given. This is an unlikely requirement in the A & E department as most babies brought for resuscitation will usually have been born suddenly and unexpectedly.

3. A baby in terminal apnoea is pale, floppy, and apnoeic with a heart rate of less than 80. He may be hypothermic. The baby should be intubated and ventilated as above, and if the heart rate is continuing to slow an assistant should perform cardiac massage at a rate of 120 per minute. In neonates, the 'hands around the chest' method of cardiac compression produces a better cardiac output than simple sternal compression with the fingers (p. 16). Adrenaline (0.1 ml/kg of 1:10 000) may be given intravenously or via the endotracheal tube as described on p. 18. The umbilical vein should be catheterized. The umbilical tape should be tied loosely around the umbilical cord and the cord should be transected with a scalpel, leaving a 1 cm stump. Three vessels will now be seen. Two will be small contracted arteries and the third a large dilated vein. A fine saline-filled feeding tube can easily be inserted into this vessel and the umbilical tape then tightened to secure it. The tube should be inserted for about 5 cm. It should then lie in the inferior vena cava. Two to five millilitres of 8.4 per cent sodium bicarbonate can be slowly injected into the umbilical vein; this can then be followed by 2–5 ml of 10 per cent dextrose. If there is no response to the bicarbonate, further adrenaline should be given into the umbilical vein. Later the feeding tube can be stitched into the cord. ECG leads should be put on the baby's chest.

Action to take if poor response to resuscitation:

1. Check for technical fault.

- Is the oxygen connected to the bag system?
- Is the endotracheal tube in the trachea? Listen to the chest for air entry and observe chest and abdominal movement.
- Is the endotracheal tube too far down in a bronchus? Listen to both sides of the chest for unequal air entry.

2. Has the baby a pneumothorax? Auscultate the chest for asymmetry of breath sounds, and feel for a displaced cardiac apex and trachea. A cold light source can be used to transilluminate the chest. A pneumothorax may show as a hyperilluminating area (if this test is negative, pneumothorax is not excluded). If a pneumothorax is clinically thought to be present, a 21 or 23 gauge butterfly needle should be inserted through the second intercostal space at the mid-clavicular line. The end of the butterfly tube should be in a gallipot under saline. If a pneumothorax is present, air bubbles will be seen in the saline. The baby will improve as the pneumothorax is no longer under tension. A confirmatory X-ray can now be done and a properly placed chest drain inserted by the paediatrician.

3. Does the baby have evolving lung disease, such as respiratory distress syndrome or congenital pneumonia? If the lungs are stiff to ventilate, increased frequency and pressure of ventilation should be tried.

4. Does the baby have a congenital abnormality obstructing respiration, such as a diaphragmatic hernia? This can be diagnosed on a chest X-ray, but only supportive treatment is feasible until the child is transferred to a neonatal surgical unit.

5. Is there profound anaemia? These babies will require exchange transfusion. The procedure should be carried out by the paediatrician.

When to stop resuscitation

If there are no technical difficulties but there has been no effective cardiac activity after resuscitation, for 30 minutes, it is appropriate to cease efforts (see also Chapter 15).

Post-resuscitation care

1. Hypothermia is a major hazard for newborn premature babies. It will increase acidosis and reduce the chance of a good outcome. The baby should be dried and well wrapped in warm dry blankets. Make sure that the head is covered as this is a major source of heat loss. The baby's temperature should be monitored rectally with a low-reading thermometer. If the department has an overhead heater this will be very useful, but care must also be taken to minimize convective losses if the baby is nursed on an open surface.

2. Any preterm asphyxiated baby is highly likely to develop respiratory distress syndrome, and if there is continuing respiratory difficulty after resuscitation the endotracheal tube should remain in place and ventilatory assistance continued during transfer to the neonatal unit.

3. Oxygen toxicity is a worry in babies of less than 32 weeks. Although the retinopathy of prematurity has probably many causative factors, there is a link with high oxygen levels in the blood. During resuscitation 100 per cent oxygen is necessary and this requirement outweighs any other. After resuscitation, continued high ambient oxygen is usually necessary as there is often evolving respiratory distress syndrome following asphyxia in a premature baby. A pulse oximeter is useful for monitoring oxygen needs and a level of 95 per cent saturation should ensure adequate oxygenation without hyperoxia. Babies should be transferred to a neonatal nursery as soon as possible.

Congenital heart disease presenting in the neonatal period

• Neonatal heart disease: management

There is a trend towards early hospital discharge for mothers and babies who have had an uneventful birth. Therefore some babies may be discharged from hospital with their congenital heart disease undetected. This is because the haemodynamic changes from fetal to adult type circulation are not completed immediately after birth. In the first week or so of life, as the patent ductus closes and pulmonary arterial resistance decreases, babies with serious congenital heart disease may become symptomatic and present in one of two ways.

Heat failure The main symptom is breathlessness particularly on feeding.

1. High-output heart failure—this is caused by a large left to right shunt, as in a large ventricular septal defect, or in complex heart lesions with an overall left to right shunt, such as single ventricle or truncus arteriosus. The physical signs are of a hyperdynamic heart with an enlarged liver and sometimes a triple cardiac rhythm.

2. Obstructive heart failure—this is caused by coarctation of the aorta or severe aortic stenosis. The classical sign of weak femoral pulses in coarctation may not be present in a seriously ill baby with low-output heart failure.

Cyanosis The most common cyanotic congenital heart disease presenting in the neonatal period is transposition of the great vessels. These babies are clearly blue at birth. However, there are some complex lesions in which, because of a large ductal flow, babies are pink in the first few days of life. They become bluer as the ductus closes.

Neonatal heart disease: management

The paediatrician should be called urgently for any baby who is in respiratory distress or who is cyanosed.

Oxygen and a diuretic (frusemide 1 mg/kg intravenously) should be given to the baby in heart failure.

An intravenous infusion of prostaglandin E (0.01–0.05 µg/kg/min) will help keep open the duct of a baby with a duct-dependent cyanotic heart disease until transfer to a paediatric cardiology centre. This drug will usually be ordered by the paediatrician after discussion with the cardiology centre.

A chest radiograph and ECG should be obtained if there is time before transfer and the baby's condition permits.

Neonatal jaundice

Babies may present to the A & E department with jaundice following early neonatal hospital discharge. Jaundice is visible when the serum bilirubin rises above 18 µmol/l. These babies should be referred to the paediatrician.

Neonatal infection

The neonate's immature immune system puts him at risk of serious infection. Septicaemia, meningitis, pneumonia, and urinary tract infection are the most serious problems. Group B *Streptococcus* and *Escherichia coli* are the most common bacterial pathogens, with *Klebsiella, Staphylococcus, Pseudomonas,* and *Listeria* spp. occurring less frequently.

Babies with serious signs, such as chest retraction or a bulging fontanelle, are clearly very poorly and will be admitted for urgent investigation and treatment. However, the early signs of infection in neonates are subtle and non-specific. Serious infection should be considered in babies presenting with the following:

• hypothermia
• poor feeding
• irritability
• drowsiness
• unexplained jaundice
• vomiting
• poor weight gain.

Neonates should be referred to the paediatrician.

The crying baby

- **Infantile colic Management of the well crying baby and his parents Admission of the crying baby**

A common visitor to the A & E department, particularly at night-time, is the crying infant with his distraught parents. The A & E doctor has two tasks:

(1) to diagnose and treat any physical illness or injury as the cause of crying.

(2) to assess whether the parents need help with what may be to them an intolerable situation.

First, a full history is essential. If excessive crying has occurred only in the past 24 hours or so, illness or injury is likely. The baby who has been crying excessively for days or weeks is less likely to have an identifiable cause. Seek a history of any symptoms such as vomiting, diarrhoea, cough, or feeding difficulty. Ask how the baby behaves when he is not crying: Is he alert and his usual self, or drowsy and un-interested? In the latter event illness is more probable. Has the baby recently been immunized? (Screaming spells after pertussis immunization are described.)

Observation of the baby both when crying and when responding to soothing is helpful in assessing his overall state of health (see Chapter 1). Examination must include all systems. First look for evidence of serious disease, such as meningitis (p. 216). Intussusception or incarcerated inguinal hernia should be particularly considered in babies with excessive crying, and the abdomen, genitalia, and rectum examined carefully (see p. 194).

Always examine the baby's ears. Otitis media is a painful disease which may cause inconsolable crying. Remember, however, that a crying baby's healthy eardrums may appear pink.

A careful search should be made for trauma, including threads from clothing wrapped around digits. Look for bruising, a painful or non-mobile limb, which suggests fracture, bone or joint infection. The baby should have a urine specimen examined as infection in the lower urinary tract may be painful.

At the end of history and thorough examination, if any doubt remains about illness or injury being the cause of the baby's crying a paediatric opinion should be requested.

However, many babies will have a completely negative examination, appear well, and have no symptoms suggestive of disease. If they have a history of recurrent episodes of inconsolable crying, particularly in the evening, associated with drawing up of the knees to the abdomen and sometimes the passage of flatus, the condition known as infantile colic is likely.

Infantile colic

This is a condition of unknown aetiology which affects babies from a few weeks to a few months old. Otherwise well and thriving babies will have paroxysms of crying with a flushed face and drawing up of the legs. In the attack the baby cannot be comforted, and sometimes relief only occurs when the baby passes a stool or wind. Theories of the causation of colic include cow's milk allergy, lactose intolerance, maternal anxiety, and abnormal gut motility. No convincing evidence exists for any theory. No medication now available has clearly been shown to be beneficial.

All babies cry, but medical help is sought by parents who think that their baby's crying is excessive. The definition of 'excessive' will depend on the parents' expectation of their baby's behaviour, previous experience with other babies, and often their social circumstances. A crying baby in a household where a parent is single, unwell, depressed, or has critical neighbours will be more stressful than one in a household with other supportive adults.

Parents have usually done all that they can to alleviate their baby's distress. Feeding, winding, changing, cuddles, and play will have been tried and it is the inconsolable nature of the crying that makes parents anxious that their baby may be ill and utterly at a loss about what to do.

Management of the well crying baby and his parents

Many parents will be much relieved by the thorough history and examination which has shown no serious cause for their baby's crying. Relief for the baby often comes from rhythmical motion—parents may have commented that a car ride has a soothing effect. The use of a baby sling so that the infant can be carried around for periods of the day is often helpful. Relatives and friends can be encouraged to take over the baby's care for short periods to give the parents at rest.

The family's GP and health visitor should be informed and asked to provide community support until the crying bouts resolve, which they usually do spontaneously in a few weeks.

Admission of the crying baby

Sometimes parents and baby may be so distressed and exhausted by the crying that they cannot go home. Admission for the baby should be offered in such a way as not to make the parents feel that they have failed. The parent may want to stay in with the baby, but without compulsion, or they may be encouraged to have a good night's sleep at home.

CHAPTER 15

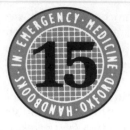

Children brought in dead

Key points in children brought in dead

1 All children brought to hospital who may be dead should be admitted to the resuscitation room and unless contra-indications are very clear, for example rigor mortis or injuries incompatible with life, resuscitation should be initiated.

2 Sensitive and caring management of the bereaved family in the A & E department will aid the long-term grieving process.

3 Ensure that all relevant community health workers are informed of the child's death.

4 Ensure that the arrangements are made for later counselling of the family.

Initial action

• The parents

Children who are found suddenly and unexpectedly dead or who have been the victims of a fatal accident are usually brought to the nearest A & E department. All such children should be admitted to the resuscitation room. Unless there is clear evidence of death, such as post-mortem rigidity or dependent skin discoloration, the A & E staff should start resuscitation. *A paediatric cardiac arrest call should be made* and it will be the leader of the arrest team who decides when resuscitation should cease.

The parents

When the child is taken into the resuscitation room the parents should be taken into a quiet room reserved for their exclusive use. Preferably, it should be near the resuscitation room. They should be accompanied by an experienced nurse who will ensure that they are fully aware of what is happening with their child. The parents' later grieving can be helped by support and understanding from A & E staff at this time.

Parents' needs

• **Breaking the news**

1. Knowledge that an appropriate medical response was made, i.e. 'everything was done'.
2. A private space and sufficient time in which to receive distressing news.
3. The opportunity to be with their dead child.
4. The services of a minister of religion and a social worker if they wish.
5. An understanding of the law's requirements in a case of sudden unexpected death. Parents should know that the coroner must be informed about their child's death. He will almost certainly order a post-mortem. A police officer will want to take a statement from them, and may want to visit the home or place of death. An inquest is usual following an accidental death, but is rarely held after death due to natural causes.

Breaking the news

Telling the parents that their child is dead is a difficult and unenviable task. It is usually undertaken by senior staff, such as a paediatric consultant or registrar, or the A & E consultant, but on occasions the task may fall to the A & E senior house officer if senior staff are unavailable.

Once the patient has been certified dead, do not keep the parents waiting in false hope. A direct but sympathetic approach is best. Make sure that you know the child's name. On entering the room sit down with the parents. The parents must be told the news sympathetically, but without euphemisms, using words such as, 'I am very sorry to have to tell you, but despite all that we could do Jason is dead'. Stay with the parents after the receipt of this initial shocking news. If appropriate and you feel comfortable doing it, you can show sympathy by holding the parent's hand or putting an arm around them. Usually the parents turn away towards each other for a while, but may shortly want to ask questions about the cause of death and what they should do now. If you are asked about the cause of death, answer as simply and honestly as possible but make it clear that some answers are not yet available.

Examination of the child

- **Post-mortem investigations for sudden and unexpected death in infancy**

The child will already have been examined during the resuscitation attempt, but any external features should now be checked and recorded in the notes together with the history.

- Fully undress the child but save the clothes, including the nappy.
- Note the state of nutrition and hydration.
- Record the child's initial rectal temperature on arriving at the department.
- Note any injuries or rashes.

Although a post-mortem will be carried out, certain investigations are likely to be more informative if specimens are collected in the A & E department. These include investigations which will indicate infection or an inborn error of metabolism as the cause of death. These investigations will usually be done by the paediatrician and the results sent to the duty consultant paediatrician who will later talk with the parents.

Post-mortem investigations for sudden and unexpected death in infancy

1. Bacteriology—swabs should be taken from the nose and throat, Stool and urine samples (suprapubic aspirate) should be collected and blood taken for culture from the right ventricle.

2. Virology—a nasopharyngeal aspirate or throat swab and a stool for culture should be taken.

3. Metabolic diseases—a urine sample, obtained by suprapubic aspirate, should be sent to the Regional Metabolic Diseases Laboratory as a few sudden and unexpected deaths in infancy are due to inborn errors of metabolism. These diseases are usually inherited in an autosomal recessive manner and the affected family will need genetic counselling. The specimen should be frozen if its transport will be delayed until the next day.

4. A small full-thickness skin sample taken with a sterile scalpel and placed in a tissue growth medium will still contain viable cells. The Regional Metabolic Diseases Laboratory may be able to identify inborn errors of metabolism from cell culture of this material.

A written record in the patient's notes of any procedure, such as suprapubic urine aspiration or skin biopsy, should be made so that the pathologist knows that the injuries were post-mortem.

Helping the family

- **Should the bereaved family see the dead child again?**
  Follow-up

Should the bereaved family see the dead child again?

Many bereaved parents find that the opportunity to sit with, look at, and touch their dead child in the A & E department makes the reality of death more concrete, and in the long run aids the process of coming to terms with their loss. Parents should be actively and sympathetically encouraged to see their dead child. The child's body should be dressed in his own clothes again and placed in a room where his parents may sit with him undisturbed. At this stage they may wish to be completely alone with their child, but the nurse who has been with them throughout should remain nearby. The parents may want older brothers and sisters and other relatives to be present as well.

Eventually the parents should be ready to go home. The nurse or social worker should ensure that there is someone from their family or neighbourhood who is able to accompany them. If this is not the case, the social worker will usually take the parents home.

A few Polaroid photographs of the child may be taken by staff. They should be carefully labelled with the baby's name and the date. Occasionally, parents later tell their bereavement counsellor of their regret that they do not have a photograph of their baby. These photographs may then be welcomed. Hair or palmprints and footprints are sometimes also offered.

The A & E doctor should make sure that the GP and health visitor are informed promptly, by telephone, of the child's death and know what the parents have been told. The GP will probably want to visit the home later on. If the mother has been breast-feeding, he may prescribe a lactation suppressant such as bromocriptine mesylate. A check-list (Table 15.1) is useful for ensuring that no detail is forgotten. Occasionally, as the result of a case of fatal meningococcal disease, prophylaxis should be given to the immediate family (see p. 219).

Follow-up

Some days or weeks later the parents should meet with the consultant paediatrician. The consultant will then have information from the post-mortem and other tests about the cause of the child's death and its implications for the family.

The family should be offered contact with a bereavement counsellor. Depending on local arrangements, this may be a hospital bereavement counsellor, a social worker who has had counselling training, a member of the Foundation for the Study of Infant Deaths (telephone number 0171–235–1721), a

Table 15.1 • Check list for sudden infant deaths

Child's name . . . . .

Date of birth . . . . .   Date of death . . . . .

1.	Registrar or consultant spoken to parents	. . . . .
2.	Brief clinical history taken	. . . . .
3.	Examination/investigations done	. . . . .
4.	Parents offered to be with/hold baby	. . . . .
5.	Coroner informed	. . . . .
6.	Medical social worker informed	. . . . .
7.	GP informed	. . . . .
8.	Health visitor informed	. . . . .
9.	Minister of religion contacted	. . . . .
10.	Advice on registration and funeral given	. . . . .
11.	Pamphlet from SIDS Foundation given	. . . . .
12.	Phone number of local Friends of SIDS given	. . . . .
13.	Consultant follow-up arranged	. . . . .
14.	Social work follow-up arranged	. . . . .
15.	Community physician informed	. . . . .

member of the Compassionate Friends, the patient's own minister of religion, or the GP.

Causes of sudden unexpected death in children

- **Cot deaths   Follow-up of siblings**

- Sudden, unexpected death in infancy (cot death)—including sudden infant death syndrome (SIDS).
- Major trauma, for example road traffic accident, fires, choking, drowning, falls from a height, non-accidental injury, or poisoning.
- Sudden overwhelming infection, for example meningococal septicaemia, epiglottitis, myocarditis, peritonitis, etc.
- Sudden deterioration in a chronic condition such as asthma, epilepsy, diabetes, or heart disease.

Cot deaths

Cot deaths are sudden unexpected deaths in infants between the ages of one week and one year. The incidence was one in 450 live births but is dropping generally. Advice to parents about placing their child in the supine position has reduced the death rate by more than 50 per cent. In the age group concerned, cot death is the most common cause of death. Cot deaths occur more frequently in the winter months than the summer months. Boys are at greater risk than girls, and babies who have been preterm, one of twins, or had apnoeic spells in the first week of life are more vulnerable. Statistically, more of these deaths occur in families where the mother is young unmarried, a smoker, had inadequate antenatal care, and was poorly educated. However, cot deaths occur in families from all walks of life.

At post-mortem some unexpected deaths are found to have a clear cause, such as an overwhelming infection, usually pneumonia. Less frequently, there is a congenital abnormality, such as congenital heart disease or an inborn error of metabolism, particularly of fatty acid metabolism. Very occasionally, accidental or intentional suffocation is considered to be the cause of death. The more careful and skilful the post-mortem, the more likelihood there is of a recognizable cause of death being found. However, in many infants who had been found suddenly and unexpectedly dead, a careful post-mortem examination reveals no evidence of serious illness. The examination shows either completely normal results or evidence of only minor illness, such as an upper respiratory tract infection. These unexplained infant deaths comprise SIDS.

It is generally considered that there is unlikely to be one single answer to the pathology of SIDS. The current hypotheses include the following:

- an abnormality of the control of respiration
- an abnormal response to common respiratory infections
- hyperthermia, exacerbated by excessively warm bed coverings during a mild illness
- some association with the prone position while sleeping.

Follow-up of siblings

If there is a surviving twin, this infant is at increased risk of sudden unexpected death. Also, parents will naturally be very anxious about such an infant. The surviving twin should be referred to the paediatric department who should manage this aspect of care. Counselling and an apnoea alarm may be offered.

Staff distress

Following a death in the department it is helpful for staff to discuss their own feelings of distress. Staff are often helped by the knowledge that sensitive, caring, and supportive management of bereavement families in the A & E department has a profound and prolonged positive influence on the response of the family to the death.

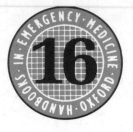

Legal aspects

Key points in legal aspects

1   If there are complaints about your management of a patient, full and accurate medical records are usually the best defence.

2   Ensure medical confidentiality.

3   Parental consent is not necessary for the emergency treatment of a seriously ill or injured child.

Complaints

Medical complaints are more frequent in A & E departments than in some other hospital departments for three reasons. Firstly, the demands of an open-door service, where patients' injuries and illnesses range from the trivial to the life-threatening, can stress all staff and render mistakes and misunderstandings more likely. Secondly, the problems with which patients present range across the whole spectrum of medicine requiring a broad basis of knowledge and experience from doctors who may be relatively inexperienced. Thirdly, patients and their relatives attending an A & E service are often anxious and frightened. This can impede the doctor–patient relationship.

The chances of making a mistake can be minimized by keeping the following in mind:

- examine the patient properly
- ask for help if you are uncertain
- be aware of your own limitations and do not take on anything which you are not confident to do
- follow departmental guidelines if available
- only tackle one problem at a time. It is easy to become distracted by frequent demands
- make good notes

Notekeeping

The importance of making adequate notes at the time of the incident cannot be over-emphasized. Firstly, many legal cases take years to come to court or settlement, and the accuracy of memory cannot be relied upon. Secondly, if there are any complaints about your management of a patient, well-kept records can often exonerate you but actions cannot be defended if they are not documented.

It is useful to start your notes with the time and date when you have seen the patient. Note who is accompanying the child and from whom the history is taken. Relevant positive and negative features of the history should be noted, and the examination notes should document the salient clinical findings. Particular note should be made of describing the absence of a relevant important sign. Injuries should be described in full, stating size, site, and description of the lesion. A diagram of the injury is invaluable. Remember to note the side of injuries, and to name fingers rather than number them. Finally, give a diagnosis, describe the treatment ordered, and the eventual disposal of the patient. Always sign the notes, and also print your name if the signature is illegible. A new act, the *Access to Health Records Act 1990*, came into force in November 1991. This establishes a right of access by patients to health records held manually, and provides for the correction of inaccurate health records. In the case of a child patient, a person with parental responsibility may apply for access to the record either if the child has consented or (in the case of a child incapable of understanding) if the access is in the child's best interests.

Confidentiality

In a busy department if it sometimes difficult to ensure the patient's privacy. Medical records may be left in different parts of a department awaiting procedures, and confidentiality may be breached. It is important to keep in mind the patient's rights to privacy.

Information about the child can be disclosed to medical and paramedical colleagues who need to be aware of the clinical findings, for example GPs, dentists, physiotherapists, etc. There is also a statutory requirement to disclose information in certain cases, for example notification of infectious diseases and notification of births and deaths.

In the case of a child attending without a parent, the parent should usually be informed of the details of the child's visit to the hospital. This may be done by relatives or school teachers who have come with the child. Occasionally, an older child may request that the parents are not informed. In this case the GP and a senior doctor should be consulted and a decision made as to whether the information can justifiably be withheld.

Difficulties may arise in relation to police requests for information. The doctor has a duty to the patient of confidentiality, but also a social obligation to the community. Information should not be released to the police without signed informed consent from the patient or parents. However, in serious cases social responsibility may override the need for confidentiality and information can be released to the police. In this case, first ask for senior advice or call the Medical Defence Union or Medical Protection Society.

As A & E departments are becoming computerized, users must be aware of the *Data Protection Act*. If medical information is held on a computer file, the patient has a right to see that information unless some part of it is thought necessary to be withheld from him. This decision is taken by the consultant in charge of the case.

Consent to treatment

Consent may be implied or expressed. In most cases in the A & E department implied consent is given by adults on behalf of children by bringing them for treatment and allowing procedures to be undertaken after due explanation. Express written consent should be obtained, after an adequate explanation, for any procedure requiring general or regional anaesthetic.

Consent may be made on behalf of the child by a parent or other adult *in loco parentis*, such as a teacher, relative, or adult friend.

Sometimes children attend A & E departments without any accompanying adult. It is sensible to attempt to contact the parents before examining and treating the child. However, if the child has a sufficient understanding of what is proposed, he may consent to a doctor making an examination and giving treatment. The doctor must be satisfied that any such child has a sufficient understanding of what is involved in the treatment which is proposed. A full written note should be made of the factors taken into account by the doctor in making his assessment of the child's capacity to give a valid consent. In practical terms this usually means that children over 12 years old can have minor treatments performed, such as minor wound care. However, for radiographic investigations and drug treatment an adult responsible for the patient should be contacted. Consent over the telephone may be acceptable, but this must be written on the A & E record. Sometimes the social work department or police can be helpful in locating a parent.

In an emergency, if a child is seriously ill and needs urgent life-saving treatment and investigations, these can proceed without parental consent. Any immediate action which is necessary to preserve life or to prevent a serious and immediate danger to the patient or other people can be undertaken. The treatment should be sufficient to bring the emergency to an end.

There may be situations when a parent refuses to allow certain treatments or procedures to be performed (for example blood transfusion in a Jehovah's Witness). Senior help should be obtained and, if necessary, the consultant and social services department would attempt to make the child a ward of court.

For children who are in the care of the local authority, the relevant social services department is able to give consent to treatment.

Child abuse

' The *Children and Young Persons Act 1933* made it a criminal offence for anyone over 16 who has the custody, charge, or care of a child under 16 wilfully to ill treat, neglect, or abandon that child, or expose him or her to unnecessary suffering or injury to health.

If a child is thought to have been physically or mentally abused, sexually assaulted, or neglected, the perpetrator can be prosecuted under the above law. It may be necessary for the child to be removed from his home to a place of safety, which may be a hospital or a foster home, for his own protection until the full details of the case can be assessed. A *Place of Safety Order* would then be obtained from a magistrate by the social services department or the police.

Section 28 (1) of the Children and Young Person's Act 1969 gives authority to a Justice:

to detain the child in a place of safety if there is a reasonable cause to believe that his/her proper development is being avoidably prevented or neglected or his/her health is being avoidably impaired or neglected or he/she is being ill-treated.

A new wide ranging act, the *Children's Act 1989* came into force in October 1991 and supersedes the previous acts. As far as child protection is concerned, the new act emphasizes partnership with parents and aims at the prevention of abuse. However, immediate power to intervene to protect children is given in the *Emergency Protection Order*, which enables a child to b made safe when he or she may otherwise suffer harm. Anyone may apply to the court for such an order on behalf of a child, although it will usually be obtained by a local authority. The order lasts for a maximum of eight days.

Police statements

You may be asked by the police to provide a statement about the injuries sustained by a patient whom you have seen in the A & E department. It is necessary to obtain consent from the patient or parent, as appropriate, to release such details, and the police will usually already have obtained this. A police statement is a statement of fact and should only contain information which you yourself can verify, i.e. physical findings. No mention should be made of the history, which is hearsay. Never dictate a statement to a policeman but write it yourself, or if possible have it types and check it carefully. Ask your consultant for advice if you have any problems. Always keep a copy of the statement and your A & E notes in case you are asked to appear in court. A fee is usually paid for a police statement.

Giving evidence in court

If a case later comes to court, you may be asked to appear as a professional witness. This does not happen often, as usually your police statement will suffice. As a witness you will be called into court and guided to the witness box. You will be asked to swear on oath or an affirmation. The first few questions will be your name, address, and occupation. You will then be asked to give a factual account of the patient's injuries. Direct your answers to the Bench. You may refer to your notes, but ask the court's permission first. You should not give any opinion as to the causation of the injuries, as such opinions should only be provided by someone of experience who would be called as an expert witness.

It is unlikely for an A & E senior house officer to be required to attend court in a case of child abuse as this role will probably be taken by the paediatrician. However, the A & E senior house officer might be invited to a case conference.

Further reading

1. Gee, D. J. and Mason, J. K. (1990). *The courts and the doctor.* Oxford University Press.
2. Livesey, B. (1988). *Giving evidence in court.* British Association for the Study and Prevention of Child Abuse and Neglect. Rochdale.

Index